T0299945

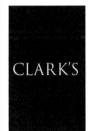

CLARK'S

ESSENTIAL GUIDE TO

MOBILE AND THEATRE IMAGING

This easy-to-understand pocketbook in the highly respected Clark's stable of diagnostic imaging texts is an invaluable tool for student and practising radiographers, providing practical guidance to undertaking a wide range of mobile and theatre imaging examinations in multiple locations – different theatre environments, the Emergency Department, Intensive Care Units, including Neonatal Intensive Care Units, and on general wards.

Carrying out examinations outside the imaging suite can be particularly challenging, given the circumstances in which they are often requested, the condition of the patient and the complexity of the environment. Additionally, management of the team and area from a radiation protection point of view is the responsibility of the radiographer and requires excellent communication skills.

Clark's Essential Guide to Mobile and Theatre Imaging takes the systematic approach adopted within books in the Clark's family and is designed to be clear and consistent, in which each imaging location is explored, the challenges of each identified and possible solutions presented. A wide range of theatre procedures is included, as well as the imaging requirements of each, and common theatre practices, such as time out, are considered.

Clark's
Companion
Essential Guides

Series Editor
A. Stewart Whitley

Clark's Essential PACS, RIS and Imaging Informatics
Alexander Peck

**Clark's Essential Physics in Imaging for Radiographers,
Second Edition**
Ken Holmes, Marcus Elkington, Phil Harris

Clark's Essential Guide to Clinical Ultrasound
Jan Dodgeon, Gill Harrison

Clark's Essential Guide to Mammography
Claire Borrelli, Claire Mercer

Clark's Pocket Handbook for Radiographers, Third Edition
*A. Stewart Whitley, Charles Sloane, Gail Jefferson, Ken Holmes,
Craig Anderson*

Clark's Essential Guide to Mobile and Theatre Imaging
Amanda Martin, Ken Holmes, Andrea Hulme, Helen Fowler

**Clark's Essential Guide to Operational Management and
Business Practice in Medical Imaging and Radiotherapy**
*Amanda Martin, Peter Hogg, Philip Webster, Louise Kemp,
Lesley Wright*

*https://www.routledge.com/Clarks-Companion-Essential-Guides/
book-series/CRCCLACOMESS*

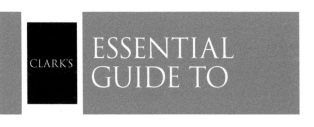

MOBILE AND THEATRE IMAGING

Amanda Martin
Radiography Consultant and Lecturer, University of Cumbria, UK

Ken Holmes
Retired Lecturer, University of Cumbria, UK

Andrea Hulme
Lead Paediatric Radiographer,
Royal Manchester Children's Hospital, UK

Helen Fowler
Surgical Clinical Education Specialist, UK

Illustrated by Ruth Eaves

Series Editor for *Clark's Companion Essential Guides:*
A. Stewart Whitley
Radiology Advisor, UK Radiology Advisory Services, Preston,
Lancashire, UK and Former Director of Professional Practice,
International Society of Radiographers and Radiological
Technologists (ISRRT)

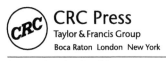

CRC Press
Taylor & Francis Group
Boca Raton London New York

CRC Press is an imprint of the
Taylor & Francis Group, an **informa** business

Designed cover image: Authors' own.

First edition published 2025
by CRC Press
2385 NW Executive Center Drive, Suite 320, Boca Raton, FL 33431

and by CRC Press
4 Park Square, Milton Park, Abingdon, Oxon, OX14 4RN

CRC Press is an imprint of Taylor & Francis Group, LLC

ISBN: 9781032147918 (hbk)
ISBN: 9781032147826 (pbk)
ISBN: 9781003241126 (ebk)

DOI: 9781003241126

Typeset in Linotype Berling LT Std
by Evolution Design & Digital

CONTENTS

FOREWORD

It has been a delight to witness the development and publication of *Clark's Essential Guide to Mobile and Theatre Imaging*. This latest addition to the *Clark's* series of pocket and desktop books is a testament to the skills, knowledge and dedication of the authors who are key members of the radiography profession and who have at heart the desire to share their knowledge and experience with radiographers and students engaged in this area of expertise. Such radiographer involvement is pivotal in the patient journey, as other members of the healthcare team are dependent on our service.

Many of us have witnessed over the years the increased use of imaging using mobile X-ray equipment in specialised healthcare settings and environments, including the use of image guidance for therapeutic procedures. This book conveys to its readers an immense amount of important knowledge that is current, relevant and essential to modern-day mobile radiography and theatre imaging.

Miss K.C. Clark, I am sure, would welcome this important addition to the *Clark's Companion Essential Guides*, which has its origins in the 13th edition of *Clark's Positioning in Radiography*.

I am confident that the patient and all those involved in this important field of imaging will benefit greatly from this publication.

A. Stewart Whitley
Series Editor
Former ISRRT Director of Professional Practice &
Radiology Advisor
UK Radiology Advisory Services
Preston, Lancashire, UK

PREFACE

This first edition of *Clark's Essential Guide to Mobile and Theatre Imaging* is an accompaniment to the 13th edition of *Clark's Positioning in Radiography*, a comprehensive bench-top guide to radiographic technique and positioning. We considered it important to build on this seminal text and give students and radiographers access to an additional text focused on mobile and theatre imaging in a pocket format that is easily transportable to any location. 'Mobile' and 'portable' are often used interchangeably when radiography is performed outside the imaging department. Whereas both imply some aspect of transportation of equipment to the patient, portable suggests that the equipment is light enough to be carried. This text will not consider this type of equipment, which is often used in veterinary radiography and in locations away from hospital sites, such as in rapidly constructed field hospitals. Instead, it will focus on wheel-based mobile radiography equipment, the majority of which is battery driven.

Anecdotal evidence suggests that newly qualified radiographers find mobile imaging, especially in the theatre environment, the most stressful aspect of their preceptorship period. It can be challenging given the circumstances in which these examinations are often requested. The patient may be ventilated, unconscious, seriously injured or infectious. There could also be a large team of healthcare professionals and many medical devices alongside the patient. The aim of this book is to provide a practical guide to undertaking a range of mobile examinations and we have included what we consider to be the most common ones performed. We have also included a brief description of the areas in which these examinations are commonly carried out. The text is based on practice in the UK, but the context is applicable worldwide.

Section 1 includes a description of the different types and features of mobile equipment and a discussion on radiation protection and dose reduction. It also offers a suggestion for ideal workflows to ensure that safe working practices are maintained from receipt of the request to completion of the examination. Additionally, a successful outcome requires management of the imaging process by the radiographer, and the importance of teamwork and appropriate communication is outlined.

Section 2 differentiates between the mobile radiography techniques used in adults and children, as techniques differ when imaging very young children. However, there is little difference in the radiographic technique when undertaking mobile fluoroscopy examinations in theatre, so Section 3 does not distinguish between adults and children. The term 'image intensifier' has been superseded by the term 'digital fluoroscopy', as image intensifier equipment has been replaced with modern digital devices, but it is recognised that, in some locations around the globe, image intensifiers may still be used. Throughout this book, the image receptor component of the mobile fluoroscopy unit will be referred to as the detector and the machine will be referred to as the mobile fluoroscopy machine.

Amanda Martin
Ken Holmes
Andrea Hulme
Helen Fowler

ACKNOWLEDGEMENTS

This book would not have been possible without the assistance of many colleagues. We would like to thank Paul Messer, Medical Photographer, for his support in producing many of the excellent photographs used throughout the book. His patience while we set up for the relevant technique was amazing, and his skill in taking just the right picture is outstanding.

Student radiographers from the University of Cumbria and the University of Salford offered their time to pose for photographs. This has allowed us to better demonstrate technique, especially in the theatre setting when the patient and machine are likely to be obscured by theatre drapes, making their position difficult to see on a photograph. Senior Radiographers Gabrielle Hart and Samantha Mahgoub from Bolton NHS Foundation Trust were outstanding in making sure that the staging of the photographs was an accurate representation of the imaging technique protocols being demonstrated. In addition, we are grateful to those patients who consented to us taking photographs for the purpose of teaching. To ensure that patient care, privacy and dignity were not compromised, some photographs were taken with clothing in place, which would normally be removed. The photographs taken on Neonatal Intensive Care Units were taken with the baby in the 'nest', which is a support to maintain arm and leg position while being cared for. If possible, this should be removed before imaging.

In addition, other radiographers have contributed to the writing, with Steven Brown helping with the imaging locations and Rizwan Rashid and Julian Booth helping with some of the theatre technique. Teaching images have also been contributed by several people and we are extremely grateful for this.

ABBREVIATIONS

ACDF	anterior cervical discectomy and fusion
ACR	American College of Radiology
ALARA	as low as reasonably achievable
ALARP	as low as reasonably practicable
AP	antero-posterior
ATLS	Advanced Trauma Life Support
BMI	body mass index
CR	computed radiography
CsI	caesium iodide
CT	computed tomography
DAP	dose-area product
DDI	detector dose indicator
DDR	direct digital radiography
DHS	dynamic hip screw
DR	digital radiography
DRL	diagnostic reference level
ECG	electrocardiogram
ED	Emergency Department
EI	exposure index
ERCP	endoscopic retrograde cholangiopancreatography
EVAR	endovascular aneurysm repair
FFP3	filtering face piece
fps	frames per second
FRD	focus-to-receptor distance
GI	gastrointestinal
IAEA	International Atomic Energy Agency
ICD	implantable cardioverter defibrillator
ICRP	International Commission on Radiation Protection
ICU	Intensive Care Unit
IM	intramedullary
IPC	infection prevention and control
IR(ME)R	Ionising Radiation (Medical Exposure) Regulations
K-wire	Kirschner wire

LAO	left anterior oblique
LISS	less invasive stabilisation system
MPE	medical physics expert
MRI	magnetic resonance imaging
MRSA	methicillin-resistant *Staphylococcus aureus*
MUA	manipulation under anaesthetic
NEC	necrotising enterocolitis
NG	nasogastric
NICU	Neonatal Intensive Care Unit
NJ	nasojejunal
ORIF	open reduction with internal fixation
PA	postero-anterior
PACS	picture archiving and communication system
PCNL	percutaneous nephrolithotomy
PFNA	proximal femoral nailing anti-rotation
PHILOS	proximal humeral internal locking system
PLIF	posterior lumbar interbody fusion
PPE	personal protective equipment
PSIF	posterior spinal instrumentation and fusion
RAO	right anterior oblique
SCBU	Special Care Baby Unit
SUFE	slipped upper femoral epiphysis
SVC	superior vena cava
TAT	trans-anastomotic nasogastric tube
TEVAR	thoracic endovascular aneurysm repair
UAC	umbilical arterial catheter
UVC	umbilical venous catheter
WHO	World Health Organization

SECTION 1
KEY ASPECTS OF MOBILE IMAGING

1. INTRODUCTION TO MOBILE IMAGING

The objective of diagnostic imaging is to produce images of optimum quality for diagnosis and to aid in the management of the patient. Most imaging is performed in the imaging department using static equipment, with access to positioning aids and with colleagues close by should assistance be required. Imaging in locations outside the imaging department can bring its challenges and is a known cause of worry to some newly qualified radiographers.[1] The environment may be unfamiliar and although the equipment is 'mobile' it is generally harder to position in relation to the imaging receptor than it is with fixed equipment; accessories and positioning aids may be limited and colleagues able to assist are not close by. Furthermore, there may be infection risks, either to the patient or to the radiographer, and infection prevention and control (IPC) processes may differ from those that the radiographer is familiar with.

Understanding the capability of the mobile imaging equipment being used, the techniques required to obtain optimum positioning and image quality, and the required appearance of the resultant images will help the radiographer carry out their role. In addition, being aware of the different types of wards and theatres where imaging may take place and the type of nursing and medical equipment that may be encountered in these locations should help the radiographer to feel more comfortable. However, the ability to effectively communicate and rapidly integrate into the new team is key to ensuring safe practice and optimal patient care when imaging outside the imaging department. Providing the radiographer is confident in the use of the imaging equipment, effective and honest communication with the appropriate members of the team should result in a supportive approach when entering an unknown ward or theatre or doing a procedure with which they are not familiar.

This chapter will focus on the basic knowledge required before carrying out any mobile examination, whether that is on a ward or in theatre. It will introduce IPC and the circle of infection so that the radiographer can understand their role in preventing transmission of infection and protect themselves from becoming infected. It will also explore the requirements of teamwork and communication in order to safely and effectively complete an examination outside the imaging department.

BASIC PRINCIPLES OF INFECTION PREVENTION AND CONTROL

Effective IPC measures are required in all areas of healthcare, as illness can compromise the immune system, resulting in patients being more susceptible to acquiring an infection during admission, known as a healthcare-associated infection. The severity of illness in patients requiring mobile imaging is such that they are highly likely to have extremely weakened immune systems and radiographers must be mindful of this when imaging them. In addition, staff who are immuno-compromised must have a risk assessment performed prior to imaging infectious patients in order to protect their own health.

Infections can be caused by many microorganisms such as bacteria or fungi, and some have high transmissibility, for example *Clostridium difficile*, norovirus, methicillin-resistant *Staphylococcus aureus* (MRSA), influenza or COVID-19. Isolation or barrier nursing may be in place.

- Isolation nursing takes place when the patient is immuno-compromised and at high risk of significant illness should they become infected, for example as a result of disease, transplant surgery or side effects of some drugs. Isolation nursing aims to protect the patient from others.
- Barrier nursing, or source isolation, takes place when a patient is infectious. The aim is to prevent the risk of spreading that infection to others. The patient may be in a single room or in a specially designed barrier nursing facility with an anteroom and negative pressure ventilation. In situations when there are multiple patients with the same infection, for example during the winter influenza season, they may be nursed in a large bay or ward; this is known as cohort nursing.

An understanding of the principles of IPC will make sure that any patient interaction is safe for the patient and radiographer alike. This starts with knowledge of the chain of infection and the processes by which the microorganism leaves its habitat via an exit route, travels to a host and enters the host (**Figure 1.1**). If the host is vulnerable, for example very young, very old or immuno-compromised, then

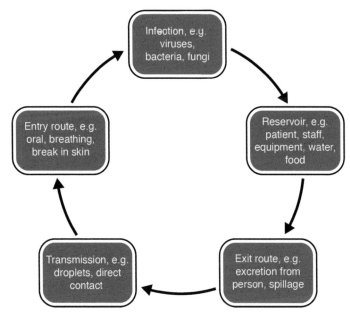

Figure 1.1 Chain of infection.

that infection could be fatal. If the chain can be broken at any point, the infection will not spread.[2] The reservoir of infection is the place where the infection thrives and can be a human or an animal or somewhere in the environment, such as water or soil. It may leave the reservoir through an exit route, of which there are many in humans, and be transmitted to the host in different ways. Direct transmission is through direct contact between the reservoir and the host, and this could be through skin-on-skin contact or exposure to droplets expelled from the reservoir through coughing or sneezing, when droplets travel directly from reservoir to host without any intermediary contact. Indirect transmission involves contact with infection that is present in an intermediary contact, such as faeces, vomit or blood, as well as on radiology equipment, in food or water, or suspended in the air on dust particles. Once the infection reaches the host, it will enter through a route often not dissimilar to the one through which it exited the

5

reservoir, such as the airways for influenza and the gastrointestinal system for norovirus.

Breaking that chain of infection is essential in stopping the spread, and there are numerous opportunities to do this:

- treating the infection within the reservoir;
- managing the exit route;
- preventing the mode of transmission from being effective;
- protecting the entry route;
- reducing the sensitivity of the host.

Many of these are addressed through effective hand hygiene (**Figure 1.2**), efficient use of personal protective equipment (PPE) and adequate and effective cleaning using appropriate cleaning agents.

Hand hygiene is critical in the prevention of infection transmission, as the hands are the main pathway for passing infection from one person to another.[3] Hands must be cleaned using soap and water before and after every patient interaction and that may include touching the patient or their surroundings such as bed linen. In some instances, they must be cleaned during the patient interaction, for example if they

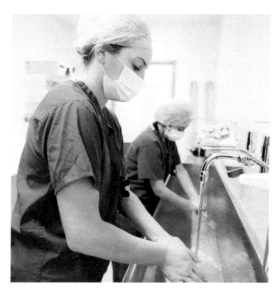

Figure 1.2 Effective hand washing is key to reducing transmission of infection.

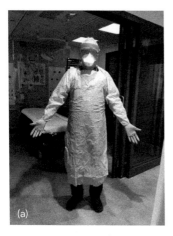 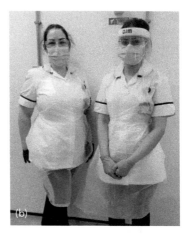

Figure 1.3 Examples of PPE, including (a) full-body protection for high-risk procedures and (b) PPE for lower-risk procedures.

become soiled during a procedure or if a sterile technique is being carried out and there is a risk that sterility will be compromised. Hands must be cleaned in a way that ensures that as many pathogens as possible are removed, and the standard process for this is the seven-step washing technique as described by the World Health Organization:[3]

1. wet hands and apply soap;
2. rub palms of hands together to create a lather;
3. rub the backs of the hands;
4. interlink the fingers and clean the fingers;
5. clean the palms;
6. clean the thumbs;
7. clean the wrists.

Hand cleaning can also be supported by the use of alcohol gel after washing.

PPE must be worn when carrying out mobile examinations when contact may be made with the patient or their surroundings. PPE differs depending on the level of risk. If the risk of transmission is high, then whole-body PPE is required (**Figure 1.3a**), with a lower level of PPE when the infection risk exists but the risk of transmission is low

(**Figure 1.3b**). Whichever level of PPE is worn, it must be changed between each patient.

PPE comprises:

- a surgical mask or filtering face piece (FFP3) respirator if a procedure involves the generation of aerosols, such as when undertaking cardiopulmonary resuscitation or some surgical procedures;
- a plastic apron, to be worn over the lead gown, or surgical gown, which must be worn when aerosol-generating procedures are taking place;
- gloves, which do not need to be sterile unless carrying out a sterile procedure;
- eye protection (protective glasses, goggles or face shield) if there is a risk of contamination from droplets, such as those released when a patient coughs or sneezes.

PPE must be donned (put on) and doffed (taken off) in a particular way so that maximum protection is received and the risk of self-contamination is reduced. Local training must be accessed, but the important aspects to remember are that the face mask is the last element to be removed and the hands must be washed prior to touching the mask using the ear loops or ties only. Hands must be washed again after removing and disposing of the mask. A video is available at www.gov.uk/government/publications/covid-19-personal-protective-equipment-use-for-non-aerosol-generating-procedures.

Cleaning products for use with imaging equipment tend to be supplier-specific and guidance must be taken before using products on mobile X-ray machines, as some may damage the structure, causing cracks and resulting in an increased infection risk. Machines must be cleaned before and after every examination, including between patients if imaging multiple patients in one location.

MOBILE X-RAY IMAGING OF INFECTED PATIENTS

Often two radiographers work together to reduce the risk of transferring infection when dealing with a patient who has a transmissible infection (**Figure 1.4**). The contact, or dirty, radiographer will deal with the patient and the non-contact, or clean, radiographer will either operate the machine if in a ward bay or remain outside if the patient is in a single room.[4]

- During imaging, the only person to touch the patient or their surroundings will be the contact radiographer. They will use a protective cover over the detector and, after imaging, the non-contact radiographer will remove the detector from within the protective cover without touching the cover. If imaging is taking place in a single room, this exchange will happen at the doorway to the room.
- The contact radiographer must clean the X-ray machine down inside the room before passing it to the non-contact radiographer for a secondary clean outside the room. If imaging in a bay, then the non-contact radiographer must clean the X-ray machine prior to leaving the bay and then it must be cleaned again outside the bay.
- The non-contact radiographer must wipe down the lead protection of the contact radiographer prior to removal.

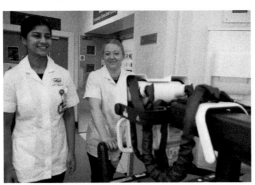

Figure 1.4 Two radiographers attend an infected patient.

THE STERILE ENVIRONMENT IN THEATRE

The risk of the patient getting an infection while in the operating theatre is around 17%,[5] with risk increasing with age, with operating time and in procedures that involve implants. The infection can be limited to a local wound infection or can become life threatening in cases such as necrotising fasciitis or sepsis. The role of the radiographer in theatre is to provide imaging support to the surgeon, but they must also be responsible for helping to reduce the risk of infection. They can do this by having some knowledge of the surgical procedure and the expectations of the surgeon so that the radiographic element can be completed in a timely manner. In addition to knowing the radiographic aspect of the procedure, the radiographer also needs to have good understanding of the additional requirements of IPC in a theatre setting. Before entering the theatre, scrubs, surgical mask and cap, and theatre clogs must be worn (**Figure 1.5**).

There will be a sterile environment around the patient, with sterile drapes and surgical trolleys (**Figure 1.6**). Movement of the machine in a restricted environment can cause it to contaminate the sterile area, so the mobile fluoroscopy machine must also have sterile covers covering the X-ray tube, C-arm and image receptor. It is essential that every step is taken so that the sterile environment is not breached.

Movement of people around theatre is also a source of infection as the air is disturbed and contaminated particles may move into the surgical site. Some theatres, including those where orthopaedic surgery takes place, will have a special ventilation system, known as a laminar flow system. A steady flow of filtered air travels in one direction, resulting in continuous air exchange around the patient.[6] Positive pressure is used to assist in this circulation of clean air, aiming to minimise the amount of bacteria in the surgical field.

It is documented that adverse surgical events, which include intra-operative infection, may occur because of poor communication.[5] Communication is key to achieving a safe and successful outcome to any radiological examination.

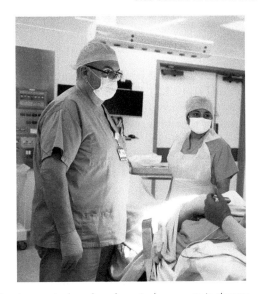

Figure 1.5 Scrubs, surgical mask and surgical cap worn in theatre.

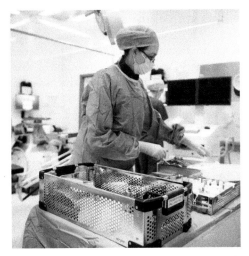

Figure 1.6 Theatre environment with sterile drapes and surgical trolleys.

TEAMWORK AND COMMUNICATION

A team can be any number of people and can include the patient if they are conscious (**Figure 1.7**). The team may range from the radiographer and the nurse looking after the patient to the radiographer and a complete trauma or theatre team. There may also be healthcare students in that team. The radiographer may work in many different teams in a single day, even imaging the same patient on multiple occasions yet working with a different team each time. However many people are involved, when undertaking imaging examinations away from the imaging department, quick integration into that team is essential.

Knowledge of the different roles in a ward and theatre environment will help to identify team members with which the radiographer needs to communicate to carry out the imaging procedure effectively and without incident. Introductions to key staff members and learning their names helps embed the radiographer in the team, as does awareness of working practices or the culture on the unit, as this demonstrates respect for their environment. Engaging with those involved in the care of the patient from the outset allows a successful outcome to be achieved, as every team member has a shared responsibility for achieving a diagnostic image. One of the key team members may not be a staff member. Paediatrics is a good example of where a successful examination may come down to how well the radiographer has communicated with the parent in order to gain the co-operation of the child (**Figure 1.8**). Similarly, when imaging a patient with dementia, more support may be needed from the immediate carer.

Irrespective of who is on the team, each person should understand their role and that of the other team members, demonstrating respect for each other. On some occasions the radiographer may be the team leader, but on others the radiographer may have to defer to somebody else. Recognising this and taking on the appropriate role will support effective team working.

Throughout all examinations, a clear and confident communication style is needed with a lack of ambiguity and a lack of jargon, especially when communicating with the patient. Most patients in theatre who have been anaesthetised with a general anaesthetic will not be able to

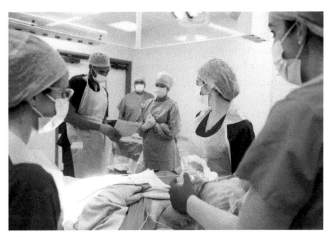

Figure 1.7 Team members in theatre.

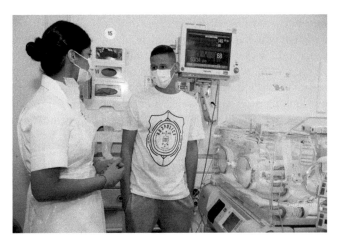

Figure 1.8 Communication with the parent or caregiver is especially important in paediatric imaging.

hear anything, but those who are having mobile imaging on a ward will be able to hear, including those who are sedated, ventilated or in a minimally conscious state after having a stroke or traumatic brain injury. Despite not being able to respond, these patients will be aware of their surroundings and therefore it is important that communication is maintained.

Communication with the patient must start with a friendly introduction, stating name and job role and a summary of what the expected outcome will be. If the patient can respond, the radiographer must check that they understand the reason for the examination. Eye contact must be maintained, as this demonstrates to the patient that they are important. It builds their confidence in the ability of the radiographer to complete the task. Watching the patient's body language will help identify whether they feel uncomfortable or frightened with a particular aspect of the pending examination. There will be instances when communication like this will not be possible and alternative strategies will need to be considered. An example of this would be when dealing with a patient who has been identified as having a specific learning disability that inhibits normal ways of communicating. Observe the reactions of the patient when entering their room or bed space, as this will give an indication of how to approach the situation. Take time to speak to those looking after the patient, such as a parent, carer or healthcare professional. They will be able to assist with identification checks and give an insight into the patient's likes and dislikes; for example, a patient with autism may not like sudden movements or noises, so a slow and quiet approach will be needed. Regardless of who the radiographer is communicating with, a clear and confident approach, with direct and unambiguous instruction, will result in a successful examination.

CHAPTER SUMMARY

- The objective of diagnostic imaging is to produce images of optimum quality for diagnosis and to aid in the management of the patient.
- Excellent IPC measures are required in all areas of healthcare to reduce the risk of healthcare-associated infections, which can be greater in seriously ill patients.
- A good understanding of the principles of the chain of infection will make sure that any patient interaction is safe for both patient and radiographer alike.
- Appropriate use of PPE, good hand hygiene and use of two radiographers will reduce the risk of transmission.
- The risk of the patient getting an infection while in the operating theatre is high and it is essential that every step is taken so that the sterile environment is not breached.
- When undertaking imaging examinations away from the imaging department, quick integration into the team with clear and effective communication is essential.

REFERENCES

1. Martin, A.J. and Dodd, E. First steps into practice: the value of preceptorship. *Imaging and Oncology* 2020;**34**:34–39.
2. Shaw, K. Prevention by breaking the chain of infection. *Nursing Times* 2016;**112**(39/40):12–14.
3. World Health Organization. *Guidelines on Hand Hygiene in Health Care.* Geneva: WHO, 2009.
4. International Society of Radiographers and Radiological Technologists. *International Covid-19 Support for Radiographers and Radiological Technologists.* ISRRT, 2020.
5. Spagnolo, A.M., Ottria, G., Amicizia, D., Perdelli, F. and Cristina, M.L. Operating theatre quality and prevention of surgical site infections. *Journal of Preventative Medicine and Hygiene* 2013;**54**(3):131–137.
6. James, M., Khan, W.S., Nannaparaju, M.R., Bhamra, J.S. and Morgan-Jones, R. Current evidence for the use of laminar flow in reducing infection rates in total joint arthroplasty. *Open Orthopedics Journal* 2015;9:495–498.

2. MOBILE IMAGING EQUIPMENT

Imaging outside the imaging department is undertaken only when the patient is too unwell to be transferred safely. There are several machines that are capable of being moved to the patient's location and these are referred to as mobile or portable X-ray machines. The terms are used interchangeably but, more commonly, the term 'portable' refers to a small compact machine that is lightweight and can be transported easily to any location by use of a carrying handle. These machines are used by veterinary surgeons in locations that are remote from any medical facilities, such as small islands, or in field hospitals, which are often set up for rapid assessment of casualties following a disaster or in a military zone. The term 'mobile' in this chapter relates to wheel-based mobile imaging equipment, the majority of which is battery-driven, which can be found in hospital settings around the world. This chapter will focus on mobile imaging equipment.

Mobile imaging equipment has changed dramatically in recent years but there may still be a wide variety of machines in use around the world. Although the ergonomics of the equipment have stayed the same, the way in which we view the resultant image has changed significantly with the progression from film/screen technology-based equipment, requiring film to be processed using chemicals, to digital equipment, which displays the image using pixels. This book will focus on digital imaging, which is in use throughout the UK. Currently there are two types of digital mobile radiography machine: those that utilise computed radiography (CR) technology and those that produce images using direct digital technology, known as either direct digital radiography (also known as DDR) or more simply digital radiography (DR). As DR is the developing technology, this is what will be focused on primarily in this chapter. In addition, there are two types of mobile fluoroscopy machine: the conventional machine using image intensifiers to produce an image and the new generation of equipment using flat panel detector technology.

MOBILE RADIOGRAPHY EQUIPMENT

Mobile radiography machines need to be ergonomic for both the user and the environments they are expected to work in. As discussed in Chapter 1, the machines need to be able to acquire images of patients whose underlying condition and status leaves them too unwell to attend the imaging department. Examples of these areas are intensive care, theatre and resuscitation bays and these are outlined in more detail in Chapter 5. These settings, by their nature, are often busy with both essential equipment and staff.

Mobile radiography machines may be manually pushed or motorised. Motorised machines are easier to manoeuvre and allow for both the small and the gross movements required when positioning the machine alongside the bed. When moving and positioning the machine, care should be taken to not obstruct those providing care to the patient. Motorised machines are driven from battery power, so it is imperative that the machine is charged after use so that it is ready for the next time it is needed. They can also be operated by battery power to generate X-rays, and this allows versatility in a variety of environments above that of a mains-powered machine, which is limited by the length of the cable required to connect it to mains power. All machines are designed to be able to fit into small areas and have either a base unit with a small footprint or one that allows it to fit alongside or under beds or trolleys (**Figure 2.1**).

The generator and exposure control panel are attached to the base unit, while the X-ray tube is attached to a column and an extendable arm. The extension arm or column normally has a range of 55–205 cm focal point distance from the floor. This enables the positioning of the tube head at various heights to facilitate accurate centring. Some machines require the tube head to be locked in place to stop it from drifting away from the centring point. Due to the diversity of patients that may be imaged with a mobile radiography machine, exposures of 40–120 kV can be achieved, with a mAs range of between 0.1 and 500 mAs, allowing successful imaging of patients ranging in weight from 500 g to 120 kg or more.

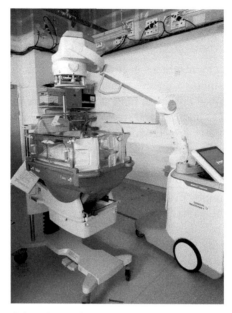

Figure 2.1 DR mobile radiography machine with a small footprint, which will fit under beds or trolleys.

Mobile machines are made of a material that reduces the potential to harbour infection and allows for infection prevention and control practices to be adhered to. Maintaining infection prevention and control is a key consideration when using detectors, as they are often used repeatedly in a short period of time on different acutely unwell patients. They are made from materials that are easy to clean with soap and water and generally have an anti-microbial coating to prevent the machine harbouring microbes and stop them from building up over time. Whenever possible, detector covers should be used to prevent bodily fluids from coming into contact with the detector. Detectors are lightweight and easy to transport around, with the newer DR detectors having a handle incorporated into their design to ease transportation.

Most mobile radiography machines have storage for personal protective equipment (**Figure 2.2a**) and image receptors, with a dedicated storage bin for CR plates or a dock to anchor and charge the detector in DR machines (**Figure 2.2b**).

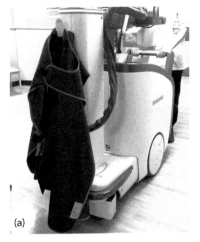 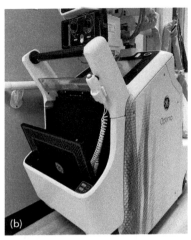

Figure 2.2 Storage on a mobile radiography machine for (a) lead gowns and (b) detectors.

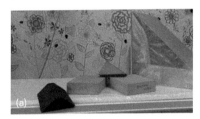 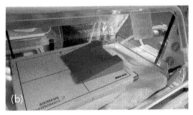

Figure 2.3 (a) Radiolucent foam pads in a variety of shapes and sizes; (b) radiolucent 15° foam pad in position for imaging neonates.

Other accessories that may be considered useful are:

- radiolucent foam pads, which are produced in a variety of shapes and sizes and can be used to help achieve and maintain the optimum patient position (**Figure 2.3**); for infection prevention and control purposes, they must be wipeable;
- sandbags to support detectors or maintain the patient position such as when undertaking decubitus imaging;
- detector covers, which can be useful to minimise detector contact with bodily fluids or other liquids; some detector covers also help to facilitate patient movement by providing a smooth,

19

drag-resistant surface that can assist the radiographer when placing the detector under the patient;

- grids, which are used depending on the area being imaged and the need to provide optimum image quality; physical grids or virtual grids may be used;

- lead back stops, which are useful when ward radiography poses additional challenges from a radiation protection perspective; local rules will outline what precautions need to be taken in different environments, particularly when people other than those being imaged may be within the controlled area; lead back stops may be used in instances where the direction of the central beam extends into another patient area that does not have appropriately constructed walls that are compliant with radiation regulations;

- detector holders, which can be used when undertaking horizontal beam radiography to help maintain the desired position (**Figure 2.4**); use of a mechanical holder also reduces the need for patient assistance, which in turn keeps radiation dose to parents and carers to a minimum.

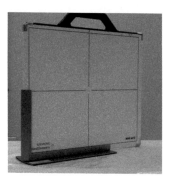

Figure 2.4 Detector holder for horizontal beam imaging.

Image Acquisition Using Mobile Radiography Equipment

As previously mentioned, images are acquired using either CR or DR technology.

Computed Radiography

CR describes the way in which an image is created using a computer system rather than using intensifying screens and film. A photostimulable phosphor imaging plate (**Figure 2.5**) captures a latent image within the phosphor layer in the form of 'stored energy' when exposed to X-radiation. The CR plate needs to be removed from behind the patient and the image is then processed away from the machine in a CR reader (**Figure 2.6**) where it creates a digitised image by releasing the energy using a laser beam. This takes around 30–45 seconds, after which it can be transferred to a picture archiving and communication system (PACS) for viewing by the referrer. The CR plate is then 'erased' using a bright light ready for the next patient.

CR plates come in a variety of sizes, which can be beneficial in a healthcare environment. For example, in a neonatal setting the incubator trays are unlikely to be designed to accept a 35×43 cm CR plate. In this setting an 18×24 cm or 24×30 cm CR plate would be a much more appropriate choice.

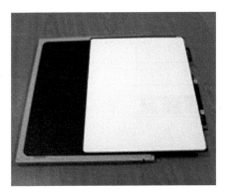

Figure 2.5 Photostimulable phosphor imaging plate used for CR imaging.

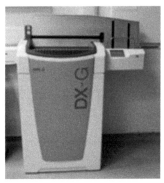

Figure 2.6 CR reader.

Digital Radiography

DR uses an image receptor, or detector, which can directly capture data digitally and process it to create an image. While different manufacturers use slightly different technologies, most rely on scintillation to create the image. Within the detector is a scintillator made of phosphor, such as thallium-doped caesium iodide (CsI), which converts the X-rays into light. The light then interacts with a photodiode array where it is converted into an electrical charge that can be digitally read to produce an image within seconds (**Figure 2.7**). Further information on this technology is available in *Clark's Positioning in Radiography*, 13th edition.[1]

The image can be viewed on a monitor attached to the mobile radiography machine without the need for the detector to be removed from under the patient (**Figure 2.8**). This saves time and reduces disruption for the patient and staff caring for them. In the event of lines or tubes being incorrectly placed, adjustments can be made promptly and the image can be repeated if required without the need for further manual handling of the patient. However, this convenience may lead to

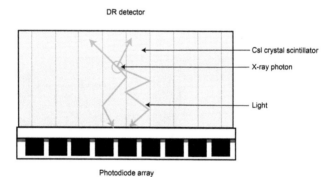

Figure 2.7 Example of scintillation technology within a DR detector.

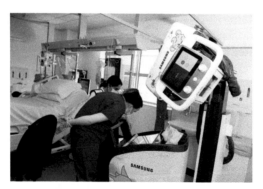

Figure 2.8 Clinician viewing an image on a DR mobile X-ray machine.

excessive exposures[2] with clinicians seeking additional imaging to reassure themselves that the adjustments made are accurate.

Various detector sizes are available; however, in a clinical setting where most of the patients are adults, a 35×43 cm detector will be able to provide imaging in most cases. Like CR plates, a smaller detector would be more appropriate for settings that also image younger patients and is essential if imaging on a Neonatal Intensive Care Unit or Special Care Baby Unit.

While technology has advanced to the benefit of both service user and provider, budgets may not have. DR equipment is more expensive than CR equipment, with CR plates being a fraction of the cost of detectors. If CR facilities are still available, the variety of sizes of CR plates offers greater flexibility when optimising paediatric imaging. However, if CR is not available, the need to image children in a mobile setting may not outweigh the cost of purchasing a smaller detector. As a compromise, some manufacturers have developed a way to upgrade conventional mobile radiography machines to enable them to have a digital capacity. This process is commonly referred to as retrofitting and allows for the analogue mobile radiography machine to be used along with a detector. The cost of retrofitting analogue equipment may offset the cost of purchasing two detector sizes and allow for greater bedside speed and efficiency but may be significantly less than the cost of a DR machine. While the image can be viewed within a matter of seconds at the patient's bedside, there is also the ability to apply post-processing algorithms to optimise the image, although this should not take preference over using correct imaging parameters.

When using a traditional film/screen technology it is immediately obvious if the exposure is acceptable or not: overexposure results in a dark image (greater density), while underexposure results in a light image (lower density). However, with digital imaging the wide latitude of the CR plate or detector, and how the data are processed, allow for the image to be digitally optimised. This means that even if the image has been over- or underexposed it may still look acceptable to the viewer. The only way the operator can be reassured that doses are being kept within an acceptable range is to ensure they observe the detector dose indicator (known as the DDI) or exposure index (EI). The terminology may vary depending on the manufacturer and, for this reason, when utilising this type of technology guidance from the manufacturer should always be sought to ensure that exposures are optimised and therefore patient doses are kept as low as reasonably practicable (ALARP). All machines should also have a dose-area product meter to allow for accurate dose recording.

DR detectors overall offer a dose reduction to patients due to their ability to optimise the image quality and their use of different algorithms without having to repeat the examination.[3]

Image Quality Using Mobile Radiography Equipment

Optimum image quality is achieved when the resultant image has good contrast and density, with minimal unsharpness and good spatial resolution. Contrast and density are controllable by selecting the correct exposure parameters, and unsharpness is minimised by ensuring the body part being imaged is close to the detector and movement is eliminated. Spatial resolution, the ability to differentiate between adjacent structures, is impacted by pixel size and is not as easily controlled, as it is dependent upon both the imaging receptor technology and the screen on which the image is viewed. A smaller pixel size will result in better spatial resolution and more detail will be visible within the image. The advent of digital imaging has affected this and it is acknowledged that spatial resolution in digital imaging is less than that of conventional film/screen combinations.[3] For most examinations carried out using mobile radiography equipment, spatial resolution is not generally a problem due to the type of examinations conducted, being of large body parts such as the chest or abdomen. These do not generally require fine detail. However, pixel size should remain a factor when selecting equipment that may be used for imaging in paediatrics, particularly neonates, in which the changes can be extremely subtle and optimum image quality is required.

Traditionally, several techniques have been used to improve image quality, such as air gaps and grids. The traditional physical grid provides challenges in mobile situations due to the difficulties in achieving perfect X-ray tube and grid alignment, often resulting in grid cut-off and thus degrading part of the image. DR, however, has the capability to utilise a computer algorithm instead of a physical grid to imitate the reasons a grid may be used to produce a viewable image, known as virtual grid software. The software uses algorithms to recreate a new copy of the image that attempts to eliminate scatter. Exposure parameters do not need to be increased as they would be using a traditional grid, thus reducing the patient dose by around 18%.[4] In addition, further algorithms are available that can suppress bone to further enhance the lungs or to highlight lines or tubes. This is particularly useful when an image may be requested for nasogastric (NG) or nasojejunal (NJ) tube position. The visibility of the NG/NJ tube below the diaphragm is often poor. By applying a software algorithm to the original image, an additional image is produced and the NG/NJ tube can be better visualised without the need for repeat imaging and additional radiation dose (**Figure 2.9**).

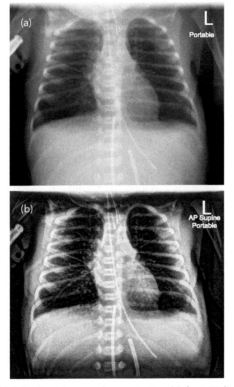

Figure 2.9 Mobile chest images demonstrating (a) the initial image and (b) the image after application of software to demonstrate the NG tube.

MOBILE FLUOROSCOPY EQUIPMENT

In the same way as there is a need to provide mobile ward radiography, there are occasions when a radiographer will be required to provide imaging in a theatre to assist the surgeon. The types of procedure being carried out will determine what type of imaging is required. If the surgeon only wants to visualise the final position of a line or a fracture following manipulation and application of plaster, this can be done using a mobile radiography machine. However, there are many occasions when dynamic imaging is beneficial (see Chapter 9), and this is provided by a mobile fluoroscopy machine. There is a range of mobile fluoroscopy machines available that provide the surgeon with support during procedures, as follows.

- Mini C-arm mobile fluoroscopy machines are smaller versions of the traditional machine. They have a reduced radiation output and are operated by the surgeon, following appropriate training, when carrying out non-complex extremity surgery.
- O-arm mobile fluoroscopy machines allow for two- and three-dimensional imaging intra-operatively and are commonly used in spinal surgery, where they have demonstrated excellent outcomes.[5]
- C-arm mobile fluoroscopy machines are the most common type in use and will be discussed in more detail below. The machines use either an image intensifier or a flat panel detector, with the latter becoming increasingly common in recent times.

Regardless of the type of machine, there are some similarities. They each have a base unit incorporating the control panel, which is touch-screen in newer machines (**Figure 2.10**). Attached to this is the C- or O-arm with the X-ray tube and built-in generator at one end and the image intensifier (**Figure 2.11a**) or flat panel detector (**Figure 2.11b**) at the other end. Advantages and disadvantages of both image intensifiers and flat panel detectors are summarised in **Table 2.1**.

Image intensifiers and flat panel detectors can be of various sizes, with machines used for vascular work, for example, requiring a larger field of view and therefore having a larger image intensifier or flat panel detector. The C-arm may differ in size and is smaller in the mini C-arm

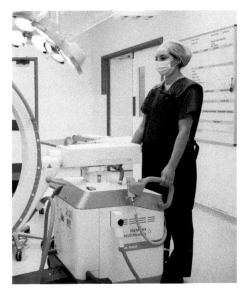

Figure 2.10 Mobile fluoroscopy machine base unit incorporating a control panel.

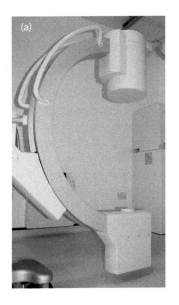

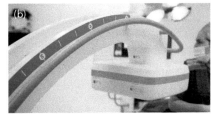

Figure 2.11 (a) C-arm with X-ray tube at the bottom and image intensifier at the top; (b) flat panel detector.

Table 2.1 Summary of advantages and disadvantages of image intensifiers and flat panel detectors.[6]

	Advantages	Disadvantages
Image intensifiers	Less expensive than a flat panel detector	Image intensifiers are bulky Higher radiation dose Loss of detail when operating at low kilovoltage
Flat panel detectors	Imaging receptor is less bulky Improved image quality by reducing geometric distortion Flat panel detectors do not use filaments; instead they use thin film transistors, thus avoiding any filament burnout issues Increased exposure latitude enables lower radiation dose	Cost is significantly higher Flat panel detectors are more sensitive to knocks and bumps and this may lead to increased breakdown issues

set up. There are a series of locks that enable multi-directional movements of the C-arm. There is also a monitor that may stand alone or be attached to the body of the mobile fluoroscopy machine. They are usually operated using a footswitch. Although the machines are referred to as being mobile, they do require mains power to function.

Like mobile radiography machines, mobile fluoroscopy machines need to be compact in design and fit neatly into the busy theatre environment. Due to the machine operating in sterile environments, the radiographer needs to ensure that the machine is kept clean and free from dust and bodily fluids. Most machines include features such as removable grids and laser localisers to help the radiographer keep radiation doses ALARP while maintaining optimum image quality.

Image Acquisition Using Mobile Fluoroscopy Equipment

Regardless of the type of mobile fluoroscopy machine being used, there are generally several image acquisition modes:

- continuous fluoroscopy enables a continuous run of dynamic imaging;
- pulsed fluoroscopy enables intermittent images to be viewed and this lowers the radiation dose;
- spot imaging is when a static exposure is made using the mobile fluoroscopy machine, but results in a higher radiation dose.

Each of these has advantages and disadvantages associated with radiation dose and image quality.[7] It is important to be guided by the needs of the surgeon but be mindful of the need to keep the dose ALARP.

Image Intensifier

An image intensifier comprises a vacuum environment with a layer of input phosphor, commonly sodium-activated CsI, which converts X-rays into light photons. The photons are converted into electrons by a photocathode and then intensified and converted back into light photons by the output phosphor. The image created is then visible on the monitor.

Mobile Fluoroscopy Machine with a Flat Panel Detector

The flat panel detector of a mobile fluoroscopy machine is a similar design as that in a DR mobile radiography machine, but a dynamic image is visualised.

Image Quality Using Mobile Fluoroscopy Equipment

The convexity of the input phosphor in the image intensifier leads to distortion at the edges of the image when imaging larger body parts requiring the whole field of view. In contrast, a flat panel detector has a larger field of view meaning that more of the area under investigation can be visualised on one image and as indicated by the name: it is flat, so edge distortion is not a problem. The internal components of an image intensifier are subject to degradation, resulting in reduced image quality.[8] Flat panel detectors have a higher spatial resolution with a wider range of densities making it easier to see detail on images.

CHAPTER SUMMARY

- Irrespective of the type of machine in use in today's clinical environment they have a very real purpose in helping support clinicians in their diagnosis and treatment of patients.
- To be able to carry out effective mobile radiography in a variety of settings, it is essential that the radiographer is familiar with the mobile radiography or fluoroscopy machine that they are using and that they are aware of the advantages and limitations of each type of machine.
- To help address some of the challenges there are a range of accessories available to help assist the radiographer achieve mobile images that are of diagnostic quality while still maintaining a low dose.

REFERENCES

1. Whitley, A.S., Jefferson, G., Holmes, K., Hoadley, G., Sloane, C. and Anderson, C. *Clark's Positioning in Radiography*, 13th edn. London: CRC Press, 2015.
2. Vano, E. ICRP recommendations on "Managing patient dose in digital radiology". *Radiation Protection Dosimetry* 2005;**114**(1–3):126–130.
3. Allisy-Roberts, P. and Williams, J. Digital radiography. In *Farr's Physics for Medical Imaging*, 2nd edn. WB Saunders, 2008, pp. 79–90.
4. Ahn, S.Y., Chae, K.J. and Goo, J.M. The potential role of grid-like software in bedside chest radiography in improving image quality and dose reduction: an observer preference study. *Korean Journal of Radiology* 2018;**19**(3):526–533.
5. Wen, B., Chen, Z., Sun, C., Jin, K., Zhong, Z., Liu, X. et al. Three-dimensional navigation (O-arm) versus fluoroscopy in the treatment of thoracic spinal stenosis with ultrasonic bone curette: a retrospective comparative study. *Medicine: Baltimore* 2019;**98**(20):e15647.
6. Seibert, J. Flat-panel detectors: how much better are they? *Pediatric Radiology* 2006;**36**:173–181.
7. International Atomic Energy Agency. *Good Practices in Fluoroscopy*. Available at www.iaea.org/resources/rpop/health-professionals/radiology/radiation-protection-in-fluoroscopy/good-practices-in-fluoroscopy.
8. Wang, J. and Blackburn, T.J. The AAPM/RSNA physics tutorial for residents: X-ray image intensifiers for fluoroscopy. *Radiographics* 2000;**20**(5):1471–1477.

3. RADIATION PROTECTION AND DOSE OPTIMISATION

Radiation protection is the action put in place to ensure a reduction in unnecessary exposure to radiation, thus minimising radiation risk.[1] Any exposure to radiation is harmful and it is imperative that every possible step is taken to minimise the dose that patients, carers and staff receive.[2] Perhaps the first thing that comes to mind when the term 'radiation protection' is mentioned is lead protection worn by the radiographer and those staff members or carers who are required to be within the controlled area during the exposure (**Figure 3.1**). However, radiation protection encompasses much more than lead gowns. It includes justification, optimisation, use of diagnostic reference levels (DRLs) and dose limitation,[3] and principles of radiation safety from the International Commission on Radiological Protection and the International Atomic Energy Agency.[4,5]

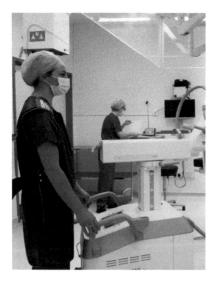

Figure 3.1 A radiographer in theatre wearing a lead gown.

JUSTIFICATION

Justification relates to the balance of benefits and risk and is conducted prior to every examination using ionising radiation. It is usually associated with the clinical indication for imaging and is conducted by the person having overarching responsibility for radiation exposures. This is generally a medical professional such as the clinical lead radiologist, although in some instances this can be a radiographer who has had the appropriate post-qualification training to allow them to justify examinations.[6] This is regulated in the UK by the Ionising Radiation (Medical Exposure) Regulations (IR(ME)R) 2017 and there will be similar regulatory practices in other countries. When the radiographer is justifying examinations, they are acting in the role of IR(ME)R practitioner.

It is usually senior radiographers who seek this extra responsibility and they generally have postgraduate qualifications, for example in plain film reporting. They must demonstrate that they understand the diagnostic value of the exposure and that they are able to evaluate alternative techniques that may have less or no radiation exposure to achieve the same outcome. They must also be able to consider the urgency of the examination and conduct a benefit/risk analysis, considering the detriment that any exposure may have. To do this, the radiographer needs to know the theory of radiation dose and the fundamentals of radiation physics and apply these to the radiation protection of the patient. They need to understand the fundamentals of image acquisition and how dose optimisation techniques feed into achieving the highest quality images with the least radiation dose. Finally, they need knowledge of the legislation, regulations and procedures and the governance associated with them. Practically, and this can be demonstrated by ongoing audit, they need to demonstrate how they use the clinical and radiological information available to them to impact on the patient pathway for both the justification and the rejection of requests. They need to be able to communicate their decision to the referrer and the patient and manage any unjustified requests appropriately.

For clarification, an IR(ME)R practitioner is not the same as a practitioner. A practitioner is somebody who practises within a profession, so all radiographers are practitioners. An IR(ME)R practitioner is somebody who has been given entitlement to take responsibility for each exposure to ionising radiation. That entitlement is given by the employer, usually the chief executive officer, after completion of the training.

Justification should address the following questions.

- Will the outcome of the examination change management of the patient? Routine chest X-rays should no longer be performed on ventilated patients unless management is expected to change.[7]
- Have previous imaging results been reviewed to see if the question has already been answered?
- Has the examination already been done? If it has, then it might not need doing again. A discussion with the referrer will clarify if this is a duplicate request or an examination that does need to be done again, for example following insertion of a chest drain.
- Is now the right time for the examination or does it need doing at a specific time or on a different day? Check that it is not a timed examination, for example an abdominal X-ray to be performed 1 hour after ingestion of oral contrast media.
- Is it the best examination for the clinical presentation? A non-ionising radiation examination may be possible in some instances. An example might be a request for an abdominal X-ray in which the diagnosis may be better demonstrated on ultrasound scan.

The radiologist or entitled radiographer cannot be around all the time to justify requests, so an alternative method is needed. Depending on local practices, radiographers may be justifying examinations against authorisation guidelines. These should be reflective of referral guidelines, which offer up-to-date evidence-based guidance aiming to help the clinician to decide the best examination for their patient. The authorisation guidelines may be local guidelines written by the person with overarching responsibility for all radiological examinations in the organisation or one of the nationally agreed guidelines, such as the Royal College of Radiologists' *iRefer*,[8] the European Society of Radiology's *iGuide*[9] or the American College of Radiology's *Appropriateness Criteria*.[10] These documents outline each examination and when it can be undertaken, as well as the situations in which it must not be conducted. They can be used in daily practice by radiographers to decide if an examination is appropriate. This is especially important in mobile imaging because the doses from mobile X-ray machines are generally higher than those from static machines, as they do not have automatic exposure control systems that terminate the exposure once a predetermined amount of radiation has been detected.[11]

When doing an examination using ionising radiation away from the imaging department there is also increased risk of exposure to those people who are near the patient. The controlled area can be harder to control and staff treating other unwell patients who are nearby may not be able to move away. Consequently, imaging using mobile X-ray equipment should be restricted to the patient whose medical condition is such that it is impossible for them to be moved to the imaging department without seriously affecting their medical treatment and/or nursing care. Therefore, when justifying a mobile examination, judgement also needs to be made about the suitability of undertaking such an examination in the requested location.

Situations When Imaging Is Conducted Outside the Imaging Department

There are several situations in which a radiographer may be required to conduct imaging outside the imaging department, as follows.

■ **The intubated patient**: a patient requiring intubation is usually found in an Intensive Care Unit (ICU) (**Figure 3.2**) and is unlikely to be moved to the imaging department for imaging, as this

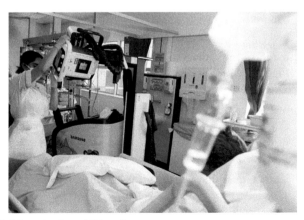

Figure 3.2 Imaging in an ICU environment.

may significantly impact on their care. They would need a team involving an anaesthetist, an operating department assistant, nurses and porters to transfer them and the equipment supporting their main functions. They may need imaging to evaluate:

- cardiopulmonary illness;
- position of tubes, lines or drains, such as endotracheal tubes or central venous catheters;
- efficacy of interventions in treating illness;
- cause for drop in oxygen levels;
- hypoxia (low blood oxygen levels);
- pneumonia acquired in intensive care;
- iatrogenic pneumothorax, that is, a pneumothorax caused by mechanical ventilation or the insertion of an invasive device.

■ **The non-intubated patient**: a patient who is not intubated may also need mobile imaging in the following circumstances:

- when the patient is acutely unwell or critically ill and that condition is unstable;
- when the patient is an infection risk;
- when the patient is immuno-compromised;
- when the patient is being continually monitored and the monitoring cannot be suspended or transferred with the patient;
- when the patient is undergoing clinical treatment that cannot be stopped.

■ **Surgery**: clearly most surgery cannot be carried out in the imaging department, so the radiographer will need to go to theatre for some cases (**Figure 3.3**). There are numerous procedures that are carried out using fluoroscopy to guide the surgeon. Examples of these are:

- orthopaedic surgery that is a planned procedure, such as joint replacement, vertebroplasty or epiphysiodesis, or any surgery that corrects a structural defect in the musculoskeletal system, such as:
  ○ trauma surgery, which is generally carried out as an emergency case. It is generally orthopaedic surgery that uses fluoroscopy to guide the surgeon for procedures such as manipulation under anaesthetic for a broken bone;

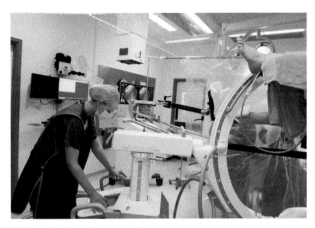

Figure 3.3 Imaging in a theatre environment.

- ○ open reduction and internal fixation for a broken bone;
- ○ placement of wires, pins, plates or rods for repair of broken bones;

– steroid joint injections, which are carried out using fluoroscopy, with injections being given into the facet joints of the spine, hip, knee or any other joint that has become inflamed; the radiographer will guide the surgeon as they place the needle into the joint space;

– urology procedures, including lithotripsy and ureteric stent insertion; occasionally these may be needed in maternity theatres as an emergency urology examination following caesarean section complications;

– general surgical cases which require a contrast agent injection to better visualise anatomy; some common examples are:

- ○ cholangiogram, which enables the bile ducts to be visualised after the gallbladder has been removed;
- ○ angiography, which demonstrates function or dynamic movement of the blood within the vessels;
- ○ insertion of interventional wires, catheters, stents or balloons during vascular or gastrointestinal surgery;

> however, this may be performed in dedicated static X-ray suites;
> - arthrography, which enables joint anatomy to be visualised, but again, this may be carried out in a dedicated static X-ray suite;
> - location of missing surgical tools or swabs;
> - removal of foreign bodies embedded within the patient.

Risk Assessment

Whether imaging on the wards or in theatre, a risk assessment associated with undertaking such examinations using ionising radiation should be conducted, generally by a medical physics expert (MPE). This should indicate which examinations can be carried out in that location. In addition, in locations where many examinations may take place, such as Critical Care Units, the MPE will have had a major influence on the specification of the materials used in construction. However, this does not happen in every location and care should be taken when imaging a patient in an unusual location. For example, a radiation risk assessment is unlikely to have been carried out for general examination cubicles in the Emergency Department. Wall structure will not have been assessed, and adjacent cubicles may only be separated by curtains or a thin partition wall. If it is essential that an examination takes place in these locations, use should be made of back stops or mobile lead screens if a horizontal beam is used. If the cubicle or theatre is next to a public corridor or waiting area, then this will need to be cleared, with somebody responsible for ensuring that nobody walks by during exposure. This becomes a controlled area and remains the responsibility of the radiographer until the examination is complete.

Fundamentally, any exposure to ionising radiation must have a greater benefit to the patient than the risk associated with undertaking it, and it must not put others at risk of unintended exposure. Communicating the conclusion of justification when the examination is not justified can be difficult if referrers are insistent that imaging takes place. Confidence in delivering the information in a clear and concise manner, with advice on who to speak with in the case of challenges, should avert any conflict and ensure that patient safety is put first.

OPTIMISATION OF DOSE TO THE PATIENT

Diagnostic imaging should answer the diagnostic question and clearly demonstrate the relevant anatomy, any pathology and any lines, tubes or hardware, such as pins and plates inserted following injury. Optimisation is about achieving this while delivering the lowest possible dose. The practitioner and the operator, to the extent of their respective involvement in a medical exposure, should ensure that doses arising from the exposure are kept as low as reasonably practicable (ALARP) or as low as reasonably achievable (ALARA), consistent with the intended purpose of the exposure. They can do this in several ways, as outlined below.

- Carrying out pre-exposure checks associated with justification, patient identity checks and pregnancy checks. Patient identification must be confirmed with the patient if they are awake. Alternatively, for the intubated, sedated or unconscious patient, either the anaesthetist or an appropriate member of the healthcare team needs to confirm identity prior to commencement of image acquisition.
- Appropriate selection and use of equipment:
  - no practitioner or operator should carry out a medical exposure without having been adequately trained in image acquisition and use of the X-ray machine;
  - the operator should select equipment and imaging methods to ensure that for each medical exposure the dose of ionising radiation to the patient is ALARP;
  - the equipment must have undergone regular, and recent, quality assurance testing to ensure it is fit for purpose;
  - the Medical Physics Department must have checked the equipment at least annually.
- Use of good technique:
  - accurate technique should be adopted to minimise repeat examinations and produce diagnostic images at the first

attempt; this includes positioning of the patient and centring and collimation of the X-ray beam to the area of interest;

– if the patient is conscious, clear instruction should be given to the patient to reduce the need for repeat examination.

■ Selection of appropriate exposure parameters in mobile imaging:

– optimised exposure factors must be used to provide a diagnostic image within the agreed DRLs for each procedure;

– copper filtration (0.1–0.3 mm) can reduce the effective dose by up to 50% and must be used if it has been determined that added filtration is required for the examination being undertaken; this is generally used for paediatric exposures.

■ Selection of appropriate imaging parameters in theatre imaging:

– when undertaking mobile fluoroscopy, the radiographer should be prepared for dynamic imaging to enable the surgeon to screen while rotating the limb or during hardware insertion; if detailed plain images are required, it would be better to use a digital radiography mobile X-ray unit as the image quality is better;

– the radiographer must minimise fluoroscopy times and minimise/optimise the radiation dose through the use of dose-saving facilities:

○ fluoroscopy screening should only be done when the surgeon indicates that it is required and has performed a procedure on the patient since the previous request to screen; an audible signal after 5 minutes' screening time will sound and this should be conveyed to the surgeon;

○ virtual collimation should be undertaken prior to and between exposures to see dose-free visualisation of adjustments to collimation; precise collimation to the area of interest when using fluoroscopy will reduce radiation dose and scatter to improve image quality;

○ pulsed and half-dose features minimise the intensity of the radiation beam; pulsed fluoroscopy allows the dose to be reduced by emitting the radiation in a pulsed rather than a continuous way; as the pulse frequency reduces, so does the image quality and an increase in the mA may be needed to achieve the same image quality;

- ○ digital spot imaging (known as 'digi-spot') is often used for final images to avoid the need for the patient to attend the imaging department for post-operative X-rays; it may also be used to obtain a diagnostic image, for example in imaging a lateral lumbar spine on a patient with a high body mass index (BMI) where neither continuous nor pulsed radiation has provided a diagnostic image; however, it is to be used with caution, as the radiation dose must be justified; prior to using digi-spot, check that centring and collimation are correct and that the image receptor is as close to the area of interest as possible, as this may show that a diagnostic image is possible without resorting to digi-spot;
- ○ the last image hold and image transfer functions allow the last image to be displayed for the surgeon to refer to and minimise screening time; unless screening dynamically, the image can be produced in a fraction of a second and transferred between monitors; image storage and manipulation allow contrast and density to be manipulated on the monitors independently after the exposure;
- ○ placing the image receptor close to the patient will reduce skin dose and magnification, which will also positively impact image quality;

■ Use of DRLs:

- – it is a legal requirement to record all exposure parameters such as the screening time and radiation dose for each patient examination;
- – doses should be regularly monitored against national or local DRLs with an investigation when the dose exceeds the DRL.

■ Continuous improvement:

- – clinical audit of technique through reject analysis must be undertaken to focus future education;

- clinical audit of exposures and doses against DRLs must be undertaken to identify those examinations that exceed the DRLs, and action plans must be developed to address the causes.

DIAGNOSTIC REFERENCE LEVELS

The employer must adhere to DRLs for each standard radiological investigation and provide guidance and procedures on how they are to be used. This is usually done in collaboration with the MPE who will assess local practice and identify the third-quartile values of the doses observed for common examinations undertaken on each piece of equipment. If the doses are similar on each piece of equipment, then one DRL can be set for that examination; however, equipment age, manufacturer and exposure protocols impact on dose and this may result in significant differences between equipment. In addition, when considering DRLs in the paediatric setting, the weight of the child will need to be considered.

Once set, the DRL is evaluated alongside the national DRL for that examination and adopted as a local DRL if it falls within the limits of the national DRL. Where local dose data have not been collected, national DRLs should be adopted. The doses are expressed as the entrance skin dose (in mGy), the dose-area product (DAP; in Gy·cm²) or both. **Table 3.1** demonstrates a sample of the minimum data required in a dose reference table.

When undertaking fluoroscopy in theatres, warning levels and notification levels should also be indicated. If the warning level of either DAP or fluoroscopy time is reached, the surgeon should be informed, and they should determine whether the procedure is near to closure. If the procedure is not near to closure, then a decision should be made about bringing in some support if the surgeon is struggling or abandoning the surgery if it is safe to do so. If the notification level is breached, the radiographer must inform the surgeon that it is now a radiation incident, and notification to the regulator is required. Local processes for doing this must be followed.

The radiographer has a legal requirement to optimise the radiation dose and remain within the DRL and, although individual doses may vary, with some occasionally exceeding the DRL, the average for standard patients should comply with the established level. When good practice is applied the DRLs should not be exceeded. The DRLs should be regularly reviewed and whenever they are consistently exceeded an investigation must take place and may involve a review of equipment performance, technique protocols and operator practices. Corrective action must be taken as appropriate. DRLs may be adjusted downwards if there is evidence that local practice supports lower levels but may only be adjusted upwards if local practices are unusual and can be justified.

Table 3.1 Examples of a dose reference table indicating DRLs.

Examination	Equipment	Local DAP (Gy·cm²)	National DAP (Gy·cm²)	Local fluoro time (minutes)	National fluoro time (minutes)
Pacemaker insertion	C-arm number 6	2.4 WL = 4.8 NL = 7.2	7	5 WL = 10 NL = 15	6
Facet joint injection	C-arm number 3	1.1	6	1.1	1.4
Neonatal AP chest X-ray	Mobile (in NICU)	0.01	None available	n/a	n/a
Adult AP chest X-ray	Mobile number 4	0.06	0.15	n/a	n/a

AP, antero-posterior; fluoro, fluoroscopy; n/a, not applicable; NICU, Neonatal Intensive Care Unit; NL, notification level; WL, warning level.

DOSE LIMITATION TO STAFF

Dose limitation aims to reduce the dose that those involved in the examination, other than the patient, will receive. It is essential that any radiographer working outside the imaging department has a sound basis for carrying out these examinations, as there is the added risk of radiation exposure to those around, especially to staff who may need to support patients during imaging.

As soon as the imaging equipment is switched on, a controlled area exists around the machine. Anybody entering this area, 2 m from the X-ray tube or the whole room if imaging in a theatre, may receive a dose of radiation and the radiographer undertaking the examination is responsible for monitoring the area. They must make sure that the only people in the controlled area are the patient and any other person who is required to stay with the patient during the examination, for example a parent of a small child or a surgeon. They must be checked for pregnancy status and given appropriate radiation protection. This may be a 0.25 or 0.35 mm lead equivalent protective apron, thyroid shield or lead glasses. When undertaking imaging in theatres or inside rooms on a ward, all doors that have access to the controlled area must display radiation warning signs and those not required must leave the area. All staff must ensure they are not accidentally exposed to radiation and have a legal requirement to protect themselves from risk. When on an open ward, the radiographer must give clear instructions to staff before any exposures are made to reduce the risk of accidental exposure. They must check in adjacent beds/bays and issue a loud warning when they are ready to initiate the exposure. All those able to move must do so, applying the principles of the inverse square law, which states that the dose is inversely proportionate to the square of the distance from the X-ray tube. The radiographer must stand at the limit of the exposure button cable when initiating the exposure (**Figure 3.4**) or, where mobile lead screens are available, these should be used. These screens may also be used as back stops when using a horizontal beam and the absorption nature of room-dividing walls is unknown.

When a patient must be supported during the exposure, the details of the person undertaking this role must be documented on the patient

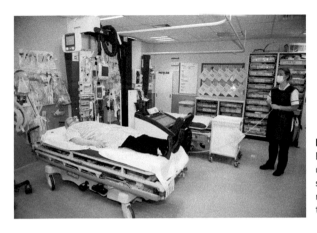

Figure 3.4
Radiographer using inverse square law to minimise dose to self.

record and regular reviews of these records must take place. It would not be unusual for the same nurse to have to remain with the patient on, for example, an Intensive Care Unit or children's ward. Where possible, rotation of staff members will minimise radiation exposure on wards that heavily rely on mobile imaging.

In the theatre environment, lead protection is available in various forms to reduce the radiation dose to staff members. Lead aprons that fit correctly and that are long enough to cover the femora should be available. They should be well maintained with correctly fitting buckles. Any staff member who is within 1 m of the mobile fluoroscopy machine should be wearing a 0.35 mm lead equivalent apron and a thyroid protector of either 0.35 mm or 0.5 mm lead equivalents. Any other staff within a 3 m range should be wearing a minimum 0.25 mm lead equivalent apron. There is, however, an argument to say that anybody entering a theatre where imaging is in progress must wear a 0.25 mm lead equivalent apron prior to entering. Lead glasses are available although not commonly worn unless by interventional radiologists assisting in vascular surgery. Lead screens are used by neurologists who may only require two images to be taken throughout a 4-hour case to avoid the need to wear a lead apron for the entirety of the procedure. Sterile lead gloves are available, but these are costly and mainly used by pain management doctors for facet joint and nerve root injections where their hands are often exposed to the primary beam.

IMAGE QUALITY

Image quality is subjective (it depends on the skills of the observer) and may be difficult to define; however, an optimum-quality image enables the observer to make an accurate diagnosis. Poor-quality images are easier to define, as they have a poor signal-to-noise ratio, and a poor spatial resolution and detract from the process of extracting information. An optimum-quality image enables accurate diagnosis to be reached. The following points need to be considered when evaluating images, as they will influence image quality and impact on diagnostic capability.

- The patient's position must enable the whole area under examination to be included in the image; distortion should be avoided by making sure that the X-ray tube is at right angles to the detector.
- Precise collimation and centring of the beam to the area of interest will minimise scattered radiation, caused when the primary beam intercepts an object and some of the photons change their direction of travel (**Figure 3.5**). Scattered photons create a signal on the detector but do not carry useful information and should be minimised by the radiographer applying close collimation to the area of interest, keeping the detector close to the patient or preventing the scatter reaching the detector by using a grid or an air gap technique. The smaller the area of collimation, the less scatter will be produced.
- If the patient moves during the procedure it will blur the image, leading to a loss of resolution.
- Check that there is appropriate brightness and contrast resulting from adequate quantity and quality of photons passing through the patient (controlled by kVp and mAs).

However, if an image appears to be of poor quality, consideration needs to be given to the reason why the image has been obtained, as it may be diagnostically acceptable. **Figure 3.6** demonstrates a paediatric chest image that is underexposed and appears to be poorly collimated. This image has been obtained to visualise an ingested foreign body, which is visible overlying the mediastinum, so it is diagnostically acceptable.

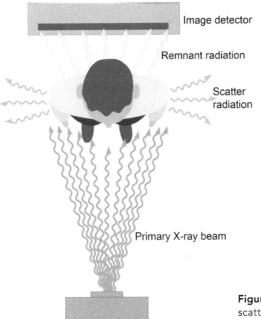

Image detector

Remnant radiation

Scatter radiation

Primary X-ray beam

Figure 3.5 Demonstration of scattered radiation, which may reach the image detector.

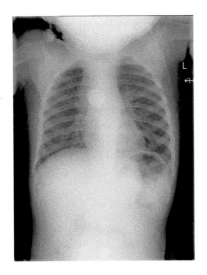

L

Figure 3.6 Chest image demonstrating poor quality, but the foreign body is visible.

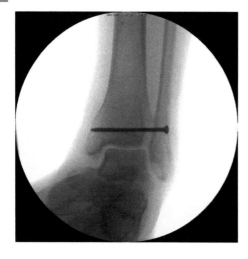

Figure 3.7 Fluoroscopy image of an ankle demonstrating poor image quality.

Figure 3.7 is a fluoroscopic image acquired in the orthopaedic trauma theatre for repair of an ankle injury. The image is of diagnostic quality, as it demonstrates the location of the surgical screw. However, close collimation would improve the image quality and reduce the radiation dose.

Finally, the steps taken after the image is acquired can also impact image quality. An image of good radiographic quality can appear poor if it undergoes incorrect digital processing or is viewed under the wrong conditions.

■ Image processing software of digital imaging equipment can manipulate the acquired image and influence how it appears on the screen. In consultation with the lead radiographer, processing algorithms are usually set by the application specialist at the handover of new equipment.
■ The display system used to view the image should be large enough to view the images at a reasonable size, be of high resolution and have an appropriate matrix size.
■ The viewing conditions should allow reduction in extraneous light and elimination of reflections on the screen.

CHAPTER SUMMARY

- Prior to any examination involving ionising radiation the operator must:
    - carry out all pre-exposure checks to ensure the correct patient is being imaged and the examination is justified, checking the pregnancy status of the patient if they are of child-bearing potential;
    - ensure that there is a controlled area of 2 m during exposure of the patient when a mobile X-ray is being undertaken, and that the local rules are adhered to during the examination;
    - use the appropriate radiation protection for the patient;
    - protect staff from scatter radiation using the principles of time, distance and shielding;
    - minimise exposure times to ionising radiation;
    - use the principles of the inverse square law, with staff standing as far away as possible from the exposed area and outside the controlled area, when making an exposure; staff should not enter the controlled area unless required to do so, for example to maintain the patient's position or the position of an instrument (the hands should be outside the primary beam);
    - wear appropriate personal protective equipment for radiation protection, for example lead gown, thyroid shield and lead glasses, if within the controlled area; lead protective shields may be used as back stops when using a horizontal beam to limit the radiation field, for example when the absorption nature of room-dividing walls is unknown;
    - optimise digital processing algorithms and viewing conditions.

REFERENCES

1. Tsapaki, V., Balter, S., Cousins, C., Holmberg, O., Miller, D.L., Miranda, P. et al. The International Atomic Energy Agency action plan on radiation protection of patients and staff in interventional procedures: achieving change in practice. *Physica Medica* 2018;**52**:56–64.

2. International Atomic Energy Agency. *Radiation Protection and Safety in Medical Uses of Ionizing Radiation*. IAEA, 2018.

3. Frane, N. and Bitterman, A. Radiation safety and protection. *StatPearls [Internet]* 2021. Available from www.ncbi.nlm.nih.gov/books/NBK557499/.

4. International Commision on Radiological Protection. *The 2007 Recommendations of the International Commision on Radiological Protection*. Elsevier, 2007.

5. International Atomic Energy Agency. *Radiation Protection of the Public and the Environment*. IAEA, 2018.

6. Society and College of Radiographers. *The Diagnostic Radiographer as the Entitled IR(ME) Practitioner*. ScoR, 2018.

7. International Atomic Energy Agency. *Occupational Radiation Protection*. IAEA, 2018.

8. Royal College of Radiologists. *iRefer*, 8th edn. Royal College of Radiologists, 2019.

9. European Society of Radiology. Summary of the proceedings of the international forum 2016: "Imaging referral guidelines and clinical decision support – how can radiologists implement imaging referral guidelines in clinical routine?" *Insights Imaging* 2017;8(1):1–9.

10. American College of Radiology. *ACR Appropriateness Criteria*. Available at www.acr.org/clinical-resources/acr-appropriateness-criteria. ACR, 2020.

11. Cohen, M.D., Cooper, M.L., Piersall, K. and Apgar, B.K. Quality assurance: using the exposure index and the deviation index to monitor radiation exposure for portable chest radiographs in neonates. *Pediatric Radiology* 2011;**41**(5):592–601.

4. WORKING PRACTICES IN MOBILE IMAGING

A systematic approach to the radiography workflow when imaging outside the department will help build confidence and ensure that all essential tasks are completed in a timely manner. The actual imaging process is only a small part of the examination (**Figure 4.1**). From receipt of request to completion of post-examination processing, local practices may differ in relation to preferred imaging technique. However, there are national and international regulations associated with the use of ionising radiation for medical purposes and they must not be deviated from.

This chapter will focus on the ideal workflow for undertaking mobile and theatre radiography. Some elements may differ from local practice, but essentially the same overarching workflow principles exist across all regions and, indeed, all countries.

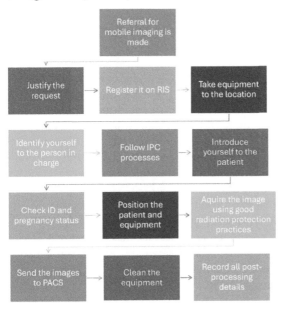

Figure 4.1 Typical high-level workflow for all mobile examinations. IPC, infection prevention and control; PACS, picture archiving and communication system; RIS, radiology information system.

MOBILE RADIOGRAPHY WORKFLOW

Receipt of Request

1. On receiving the request for a mobile examination, checks must be made to make sure that the exposure to ionising radiation is appropriate.

    – Make sure that the person raising the request is entitled to do so, following local departmental procedures.
    – Ask why the examination is being requested. It will need to be justified in line with departmental guidelines.
    – Ask why the examination is needed using mobile radiography. Make sure that the reason given is acceptable for undertaking an examination outside the imaging department.
    – Ask for the patient's demographics and check relevant recent imaging history. Indicate to the referrer if a recent examination has taken place and determine whether another examination is required.

2. Identify the status of the patient – conscious or unconscious, mobile or immobile – as this will determine the accessories that may be needed, such as a detector slider.

3. Ask if there are any special considerations, for example infection risk.

4. Register the examination on the radiology information system.

5. Review any previous images to see if there is anything that may assist in the examination, such as hyperinflated lungs indicating the need to open the collimation or a structural deformity such as dextrocardia, for which particular attention will need to be paid to the annotation of the image.

6. Gather all items that may be needed while undertaking the examination. This may include personal protective equipment (PPE) such as lead gowns and personal face masks (**Figure 4.2**).

7. Select the most appropriate mobile X-ray unit. It is recommended that dedicated units are used in some locations, such as Neonatal Intensive Care Units (NICUs).

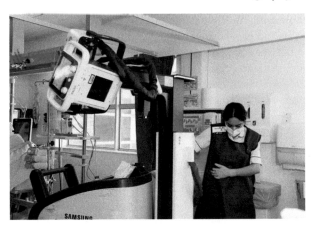

Figure 4.2 Radiographer preparing for mobile imaging with mask, gloves and lead gown.

Arriving on the Ward

1. On arrival on the ward, the radiographer must identify the nurse looking after the patient and introduce themselves, making final checks on patient status.
2. Clean the machine and the detector with an appropriate cleaning solution before going to the patient's bedside. Equipment may be wheeled over dust-absorbent mats at the entrance of some Critical Care Units.
3. Identify the patient and make an initial assessment about any support required to carry out the examination safely. Ask for this support before setting up the equipment for the examination.
4. Follow infection prevention and control measures, including washing hands, applying alcohol gel and donning PPE, as needed for the examination. Such PPE may include:

   - gown or disposable plastic apron;
   - eye protection – safety glasses, visors or goggles;
   - face mask – ranging from surgical mask to fully fitted filtering medical respirator;
   - overshoes;
   - disposable gloves.

When imaging multiple patients, it is important that PPE, such as aprons and gloves, are changed and hands are washed and gelled between patients. The X-ray machine must also be cleaned between patients. A number of speciality wards use different coloured aprons in each patient bay as a prompt to confine the use of aprons to a specific patient.

Pre-exposure Checks

Several checks are required at the patient bedside before the examination can proceed. Communication must be clear, concise and without the use of jargon. The patient must be the focus of all conversation, unless this is not possible due to their condition, in which case the most appropriate person looking after the patient must be involved in the pre-exposure checks.

1. The radiographer must introduce themselves to the patient on approaching their bedside, indicating their name and job role and the reason for them being there, checking that the patient understands and consents to the examination.
2. The identity of the patient must be checked by the person responsible for the exposure immediately prior to the examination taking place and following departmental identification procedures. This must be done against the request received, whether it is a paper request or an electronic request. The following are suggestions based on different scenarios.

    – If the patient is responsive, their identity can be assessed by asking them their name, address and date of birth and verifying these against the request.
    – If the patient is unresponsive, their identity can be established by checking their name band and verifying their name, date of birth and patient identification number against the request. In the absence of a name band, their identity can be verified with the nurse looking after the patient, whose details must then be documented on the patient record. Verbal verification of identity must be checked with any available documented information such as an incubator label in the NICU. However, when carrying out

imaging on the NICU, nursing staff must take extra care, as such units often care for twins or triplets and there is a risk that the babies will be mis-identified.

– If the patient is responsive but unable to confirm their identity because of a language barrier or hearing impairment, then use must be made of somone who is able to communicate with the patient and obtain their details, such as an interpreter or someone who knows sign language. The name of the person interpreting or signing must be documented on the patient record.

– If the identity of the patient is unknown, for example in the resuscitation area of the Emergency Department, a temporary identity will have been given to that patient and this must be used for the imaging. The identity assigned to the patient must be checked against the request. Once the correct identity has been established, the temporary identity must be updated.

– If the details do not match those on the request, then imaging must not take place. Usually, a discussion with the referrer is enough to identify the cause of the confusion. Once the request is matched with the patient, then imaging can proceed.

3. Follow departmental processes for checking pregnancy status if the examination is likely to expose the abdomen, lumbar spine, pelvis or anywhere between the diaphragm and mid-femora. Ensure that inclusive practice is followed.[1] A patient may be transgender or non-binary or may have been born with variations in sex characteristics meaning that the patient's registered sex may not be as it outwardly appears. Assumptions must not be made regarding child-bearing potential. Questions must be asked of all patients about preferred name and pronouns, as well as registered gender, in order to safely proceed with an examination. This may be done using an inclusive pregnancy status form, which can then be discussed with the radiographer at the time of imaging.

– If the patient is conscious and responsive, they must be asked if there is a possibility of them being pregnant if they indicated that their assigned sex at birth was female. If they indicate that they are not pregnant, the examination can proceed. If they are unsure, then the first day of their last period must be ascertained. If their period is not overdue, proceed with the examination. If their period is overdue or if the patient says that they are pregnant, consult the referrer who must indicate whether the examination is to go ahead. If the examination warrants fetal exposure, every effort must be made to minimise the dose to the fetus.

– If the patient is conscious but unable to respond due to a language barrier, consider using an interpreter. If an immediate means of interpretation is not available, the nursing team may have conducted a pregnancy test already. If this has been done, and it is negative, then the examination can proceed. Documentation needs to be made to reflect the negative pregnancy test. If a test has not been done, consult the referrer who must indicate whether the examination is to go ahead.

– If the patient is unable to respond, contact the referrer who will need to determine if the examination needs to go ahead and confirm this in line with local procedures.

If an investigation of a pregnant patient is needed, then particular care must be taken to minimise fetal irradiation. Special consideration must be given and privacy must be ensured when children over the age of 10 years are asked questions about pregnancy. If a child or vulnerable adult indicates that they may be pregnant, a safeguarding concern must be raised.

4. Make sure that the clinical details on the request are correct; for example, if the request states that the patient has a chest drain and the patient does not have a chest drain, then the examination must not go ahead until clarification has been sought.

Carrying out the Imaging Procedure

1. If the patient has electrocardiogram (ECG) leads applied, or anything else that may appear as an artefact on the image, seek guidance before they are removed. If ECG leads cannot be removed fully, the leads must be moved to the side (**Figure 4.3a**)

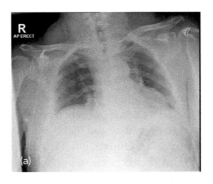

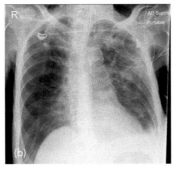

Figure 4.3 Chest images demonstrating (a) leads moved from the region of interest and (b) leads overlying the region of interest.

to avoid obscuring the lung area in a chest X-ray whenever possible (**Figure 4.3b**).
2. Position the patient, referring to the guidance in Section 2 of this volume but following these basic principles.

- Maintain open communication channels throughout the examination so that the patient and anybody supporting the patient knows what to expect. Explain each step in the process, as this leads to greater compliance.
- Minimise discomfort for the patient by doing the following before positioning the detector:

- o issue lead gowns to those who may need to stay with the patient, checking pregnancy status if necessary;
- o set up the mobile X-ray machine and move the tube head into the approximate position for imaging to take place;
- o check that everybody who needs to move out of the controlled area can move when you are ready;
- o position the detector and make final adjustments to the tube head and collimation. Detectors can be covered with plastic sheets or clean pillowcases to protect both patient and the detector itself. When using digital radiography, where there are multiple detectors available for selection, ensure the correct detector is selected and active.

3. Speaking loudly and clearly, indicate that an X-ray is about to take place. Make sure that everybody who does not need to be in the controlled area has moved to a safe distance.
4. Give good, clear instructions to the patient prior to exposure. If the patient cannot follow instructions, the radiographer must be able to observe the patient's respiration and expose at the appropriate time; for example, when imaging a crying child, expose when the child breathes in while crying or observe the abdomen for distending on inspiration.
5. Immediately prior to exposure make a final check that all non-essential staff are away from the controlled area. Consider the treatment of other patients in the surrounding areas; for example, ongoing resuscitation in an adjacent bedspace will make it difficult for those staff to move away from the area while the exposure is being undertaken. If they are more than 2 m away, and not in direct line of the primary beam, reassure them that they will be safe during exposure. Offer them lead gowns if possible and check pregnancy status of anybody who cannot move to a safe distance.
6. If using computed radiography cassettes, they must be clearly identified after each exposure and before processing, so that the correct patient information is assigned to the image.

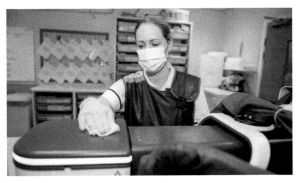

Figure 4.4 Clean equipment before and after use.

Post-imaging Procedure

1. Infection prevention and control PPE must be removed using the appropriate doffing technique.
2. Clean the equipment with appropriate cleaning products (**Figure 4.4**), following infection prevention and control methods.
3. Process the image: make sure that it is annotated correctly and send it to the local image store.
4. If the image demonstrates a life-threatening or unexpected appearance, for example a nasogastric tube in the lung rather than the stomach, the radiographer must inform the referrer/nurse in charge of the patient immediately.
5. Follow all local procedures for recording of imaging parameters, such as dose.

THEATRE RADIOGRAPHY WORKFLOW

Receipt of Request

1. Ascertain the procedure that is taking place and make sure that it is justified.
2. Ask which theatre is being used and which surgeon is operating as some will have specific preferences relating to equipment and accessories being used.
3. Check whether the patient has been sent for or if the patient is already in theatre to determine how long it will be before the surgery starts.
4. Check any relevant recent imaging history. It is unlikely that this is going to be a duplicate request, but, in the case of trauma theatre for example, it may be useful to see the preoperative images prior to attending theatres.
5. Select the most appropriate X-ray machine for the procedure that is taking place and the theatre location and make sure that all appropriate accessories, such as lead protection, are available.
6. Register the examination on the radiology information system.

Arriving in Theatre

1. On arrival in theatre, the radiographer must follow local procedures for checking in and getting changed into theatre clothing, removing uniform and any jewellery, covering hair completely with a theatre cap (**Figure 4.5**) and putting on theatre shoes.
2. After washing and applying alcohol gel to hands, the radiographer must put on any PPE that is needed. The radiographer must transfer their radiation dose-monitoring badge to the theatre clothing and make sure that it is underneath the lead gown.
3. X-ray machines used in theatre must be stored in the theatre environment and cleaned immediately prior to each case, as well as once the case has finished. The machine may already have been taken into theatre. If that is the case, the radiographer must check that it has been cleaned prior to setting it up in the position as indicated by the surgeon.

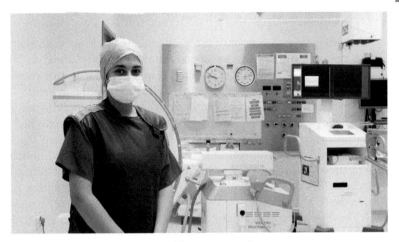

Figure 4.5 Radiographer prepared for imaging in theatre.

4. Surgical drapes may be placed over the C-arm. Not all procedures require full sterile processes to be followed, so surgical drapes may not be used, but the machine must still be covered to protect it from fluid ingress.

5. It is now common practice in operating theatres to call a 'time out' with the operating team before the operation starts.[2] This is aimed at improving safety within the theatre environment. Checks are made prior to anaesthetic, prior to incision and before the patient leaves theatre and the radiographer will be involved in these checks if they are present at the time they are being carried out. As well as confirming patient details and surgical procedure, the team will be introduced to the patient prior to anaesthesia being used. Further checks include pregnancy status and antibiotic administration in theatre to prevent infection. The radiographer present will need to state their name and occupation and they should check patient identity, if not present at the first round of checks, and pregnancy status where necessary.

6. If display monitors are available in theatre, access any previous imaging on the picture archiving and communication system where appropriate.

Carrying out the Imaging Procedure

1. The radiographer is responsible for radiation protection in theatre. The controlled area exists as soon as the equipment is turned on and it is the responsibility of the radiographer to manage this area. The radiographer must make sure that all staff required to be in the area during imaging are appropriately protected, checking pregnancy status where needed. Dedicated lead gowns and thyroid shields must be available for all staff required to be in theatre during the procedure. Warning signs must be placed on the doors into theatre and dose monitoring must be in place by use of either individualised monitoring badges or job badges associated with a specific X-ray machine.

2. Try to ensure the area of interest is in the middle of the imaging field to give the best exposure possible. Select the laser guide to help you position correctly.

3. Remember to minimise the dose by using the options available, such as pulsed and half-dose features.

4. Follow instruction from the surgeon throughout the procedure, being ready to screen for the surgeon when requested, and taking responsibility for keeping the dose as low as reasonably practicable using all appropriate optimisation techniques. The specific technique for common theatre procedures is discussed in detail in Chapter 10.

5. Local procedures will be in place for reporting the dose back to the surgeon during the procedure, as well as indicating when warning levels have been reached.

6. The radiographer has a duty to ensure the image required is displayed appropriately on the monitor so the surgeon/healthcare professional can see the monitor clearly and the image quality is maintained.

7. Throughout screening, and in particular when manoeuvring the C-arm, the radiographer must not compromise the sterile environment so care must be taken to avoid contamination.

Post-imaging Procedure

1. At the end of the procedure, the X-ray machine must be cleaned, if possible. Remove it from theatre and store it safely after sending

any images to the local image store. If it is not possible to clean the machine, or remove it from theatre, then agreement must be made with theatre staff to clean it and remove it as soon as possible, or the radiographer must return to theatre to clean it at the end of the procedure.

2. Dispose of any single-use PPE items and clean lead gowns.
3. Record the radiation dose information and ensure images are sent to the local image store and made available to the referrer.
4. Record all imaging parameters on the radiology information system.

CHAPTER SUMMARY

- A systematic approach to imaging outside the imaging department will help develop confidence and reduce the risk of an adverse incident.
- Procedures for ensuring that the dose is minimised include checking the entitlement of the referrer, undertaking robust identity checks and checking pregnancy status.
- PPE for infection and radiation risks must be used for protection of both staff and patient.
- Good, clear communication is important in conducting the examination in a timely manner.

REFERENCES

1. Society of Radiographers. *Inclusive Pregnancy Status Guidelines for Ionising Radiation: Diagnostic and Therapeutic Exposures.* London: SCoR, 2021.
2. Papadakis, M., Meiwandi, A. and Grzybowski, A. The WHO safer surgery checklist time out procedure revisited: strategies to optimise compliance and safety. *International Journal of Surgery* 2019;**69**:19–22.

SECTION 2
MOBILE RADIOGRAPHY

5. WARD ENVIRONMENTS FOR MOBILE IMAGING

Mobile radiography can take place in any location but, due to the risks associated with radiation exposure and the reduced image quality, it is generally limited to those areas where critically ill patients are being cared for. The umbrella term 'critical care' encompasses numerous locations in which patients requiring specialised care for life-threatening illness or injury are cared for, and this includes the resuscitation area of the Emergency Department (ED). Mobile imaging may also be undertaken in theatre recovery if, for example, a patient deteriorates after surgery. There may be occasions when a request is made for mobile imaging on a general ward area and careful justification of this will be needed. A short description of critical care areas is offered below.

BONE MARROW TRANSPLANT UNIT

This is a specialist unit where patients who have autoimmune diseases, immune dysregulatory diseases or cancers are nursed in individual rooms and in strict isolation. This helps protect them from acquiring infection while their immunity is lowered for the bone marrow/stem cell transplantation process. During the time patients are being treated on the unit they may require diagnostic examinations due to a change in their clinical condition. As the patient's immune system is significantly lowered, the risk of bringing the patient to the imaging department is too great. Mobile examinations are frequently requested, and radiographers need to observe the local practice in place when entering such areas and in particular the patient's room. As a minimum, staff will often require gloves, apron and mask and need to ensure the detector is covered with a protective bag to minimise the risk of introducing an infection to the patient.

BURNS CENTRES AND UNITS

Burns Centres are for patients with serious and often complex burns injuries, who are cared for in an intensive care environment by staff trained in both intensive care and burns treatments. They will be surrounded by equipment like that found in an Intensive Care Unit (ICU). A Burns Unit or Facility is for patients who do not require intensive care, but the nature of their burns may mean that mobile imaging is requested if moving them is felt to be detrimental to their care. The environment in which burns patients are cared for is carefully regulated with the ambient room temperature being tightly controlled.[1] Patients will have dense dressings in place, and this can make imaging challenging, as dressings around the torso will prevent them from being positioned in an erect or semi-erect position due to inability to flex at the waist.

CORONARY CARE UNIT

This may also be called a Cardiac Surgery Unit or Cardiac Intensive Care Unit and is where patients with significant cardiac conditions will be cared for, such as those who have had a heart attack or heart surgery. They may be surrounded by machines such as a ventilator, extracorporeal membrane oxygenation equipment, monitoring equipment and intravenous pumps (**Figure 5.1**), making access to the patient difficult.

HIGH-DEPENDENCY UNIT

This is where patients are cared for who do not need the same level of intensive care that is offered in the ICU but are too ill to be placed on a general ward. They may be attached to a lot of equipment, and will be closely monitored, but do not tend to be ventilated.

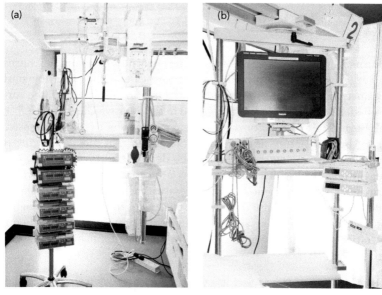

Figure 5.1 Examples of equipment found adjacent to the critically ill patient: (a) floor-mounted infusion pump stand and ceiling-mounted suction and drip stand; (b) bedside monitoring equipment and infusion pumps.

INFECTIOUS DISEASE UNIT

Some hospitals have wards that provide care for acutely unwell patients with infectious diseases or tropical infections. Often due to the highly infectious nature of diseases such as Middle Eastern respiratory syndrome or viral haemorrhagic disease, staff will employ techniques to minimise the possibility of cross infection/transmission to the healthcare professionals delivering care and others in the wider population. Precautions that need to be taken in these areas should be checked with the ward staff prior to entering. See Chapter 1 for more information regarding infection control and radiographic practices.

INTENSIVE CARE UNIT

Also called an Intensive Treatment/Therapy Unit (also known as ITU) or a Critical Care Unit (also known as CCU), this is for patients who are very ill and require intensive specialist care with high-tech monitoring. They may have been involved in a serious accident, have a significant illness or infection, or be recovering from major surgery. They may be surrounded by machines (**Figure 5.2**), and this can make it challenging to position the mobile X-ray machine alongside the bed and to access the patient to place the detector behind them (**Figure 5.3**). It often requires excellent co-ordinated team work to achieve a diagnostic image in a safe way for both the staff involved and the patient. Consideration needs to be given to the staff looking after adjacent patients, as they are often unable to move during the exposure. Pregnancy checks and use of lead protection will be needed. It is preferable to determine whether this will be needed prior to positioning the patient for imaging so that they are not against the uncomfortable detector for longer than necessary, and there is minimal possibility of them moving prior to the exposure taking place.

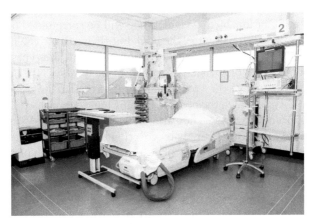

Figure 5.2 Typical ICU bay ready for a patient.

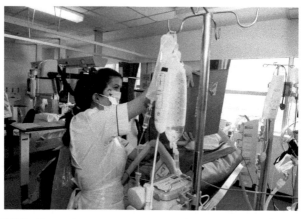

Figure 5.3 Radiographer manoeuvring around equipment to safely place the detector behind a patient on the ICU.

NEONATAL INTENSIVE CARE UNIT

This unit is for neonates who require significant nursing and medical input. Although it is most used for pre-term babies, who can be very small (**Figure 5.4**), full-term babies may also be nursed on the Neonatal Intensive Care Unit (NICU) for conditions such as breathing difficulties, infection or low birth weight. They will be surrounded by equipment, like the adult patient in the ICU, but they will also be nursed in an incubator (**Figure 5.5**). There are different makes and types of incubator, but they all play a similar role in managing the NICU patient. They help to control the environment, in particular the temperature and humidity, in which the neonate is being nursed, and keep them safe from airborne infection.[2] They also allow the nursing staff to control ambient light exposure, simply by covering the incubator, as neonates can be sensitive to light. The incubator is accessed through portholes at the side to help maintain the environment, but, when needed, the side of the incubator will lower to allow easier access.

Imaging is an important part of the neonate's care as lung disease can be life-threatening.[3] Most incubators will have an imaging tray underneath the incubator that can be accessed without having to open the incubator sides. Local practice will dictate whether this is used or if the detector is placed directly underneath the neonate. This is generally dictated by the quality of the resultant image and is dependent on attenuation of the incubator structures and artefacts caused by objects between the neonate and the detector. In addition, it can be difficult to position the neonate correctly in relation to the detector when using the imaging tray and this can lead to repeat imaging for missed anatomy.

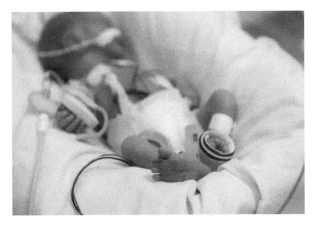

Figure 5.4 Pre-term neonate on the NICU.

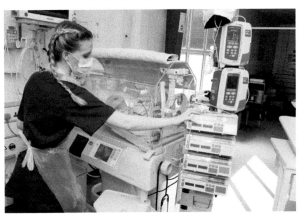

Figure 5.5 Neonate being nursed in an incubator.

This needs to be balanced against placing the detector underneath the neonate with the resultant reduction in temperature and humidity, and the increased handling with the potential to dislodge intravenous lines, for example.

Extra care is needed, as in the NICU there are often sets of multiple birth siblings who will have the same family name and normally the same date of birth, often making the only unique identifier the hospital number.

SPECIAL CARE BABY UNIT

This is for babies who do not need intensive care, but who may have been born prematurely, generally after 32 weeks. They may require monitoring of breathing and oxygen levels, and possibly feeding by a tube. There may not be in an incubator and there will not be as much equipment around the neonate as in the NICU, nor will they be ventilated. Full-term babies may also be nursed here.

THEATRE RECOVERY

This provides immediate post-operative care for patients who have just had surgery. Occasionally they may require mobile radiography prior to being transferred to their ward either due to unexpected clinical deterioration or, for example, following line insertions to check position. Imaging is frequently required urgently, and patients are often connected to multiple machines.

VENTILATION UNIT

This provides bespoke ventilation support and care for patients with severe, chronic respiratory and airway diseases and disorders, such as chronic obstructive pulmonary disease, emphysema, brittle asthma and pulmonary fibrosis. In addition, it also provides ventilation support for patients with advanced motor neurone disease and other disorders that cause degenerative muscular impairment. Patients on such a unit often require long-term ventilation. The environment will be like that found in the ICU.

CHAPTER SUMMARY

- Mobile radiography can take place in any location but is usually limited to those areas where patients are critically ill.
- Equipment surrounding the patient can make it challenging when positioning the machine and the detector.
- The incubator imaging tray can be used when undertaking imaging in the NICU, but it could result in poor image quality.

REFERENCES

1. Mullhi, R., Ewington, I., Chipp, E. and Torlinski, T. A descriptive survey of operating theatre and intensive care unit temperature management of burn patients in the United Kingdom. *International Journal of Burns and Trauma* 2021;11(3):136–144.
2. Dougeni, E.D., Delis, H.B., Karatza, A.A., Kalogreropoulou, C.P., Skiadopoulos, S.G., Mantagos, S.P. et al. Dose and image quality optimization in neonatal radiography. *The British Journal of Radiology* 2007;80:807–815.
3. Liszewski, M.C. and Lee, E.Y. Neonatal lung disorders: pattern recognition approach to diagnosis. *American Journal of Roentgenology* 2018;210(5):964–975.

6. IMAGING IN THE EMERGENCY DEPARTMENT

Imaging in the Emergency Department (ED) can be a daunting experience due to the unknown elements of the situation that you may be approaching. The patient's condition, distressed relatives and staff under pressure can all add to the challenges when imaging in this environment. Most patients are imaged in the resuscitation bays ('resus'), as this is where seriously ill or injured patients will be taken on arrival in the ED (**Figure 6.1**). They can receive intensive nursing and medical input to enable stabilisation and transfer out from the ED to a ward. Many chest X-rays are performed on unwell patients in the ED who have respiratory or cardiac disease, but the most challenging of all examinations are those that involve major trauma, that are life-threatening or where life-changing injuries have occurred. In addition, dealing with multiple patients, such as in a major incident situation, can not only cause confusion, but also be a very emotive experience.

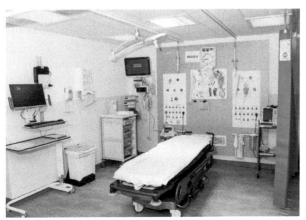

Figure 6.1 Resuscitation bay ready for a patient.

MOBILE IMAGING IN MAJOR TRAUMA

The major trauma patient may have mobile X-ray examinations performed in the emergency room, or they may go immediately to CT scanning for a trauma protocol scan. Occasionally, there may be multiple major trauma patients presenting at the same time, and a major incident may have been declared. A major incident is an event that impacts on the hospital's ability to deliver normal services.

Major incident planning is an essential requirement of every hospital, and the training and preparedness of radiographers in responding to such an incident is critical to a successful outcome. Regulation 25 of the Civil Contingencies Act 2004 (Contingency Planning) Regulations 2005 sets out the requirements for Category 1 responders, which includes NHS organisations to carry out exercises that test their local procedures for responding to a major incident.[1] Whereas the imaging department is a part of the wider hospital community and must take part in the wider planning exercises, it must also ensure that its own staff are familiar with the radiology response to an incident. The organisational major incident plan will have guidance for each staff role on what steps to take when an incident is declared, and this will include the role of the radiographer.

The radiographer taking the lead on the radiology response must liaise with the incident control room to establish the facts and instigate the local action plan, which will involve staff co-ordination and managing patient flow, as well as briefing and debriefing staff. The department should be prepared for the arrival of patients, clearing patients waiting for routine exams and making sure all equipment is available and stock is replenished. Radiographers assigned to carry out mobile imaging must make sure that all equipment is available close to the point of use. The practical element of undertaking tasks associated with imaging in these circumstances is within every radiographer's capability, but there are aspects that may not have been considered in the planning stages. The emotional impact can be great, regardless of the event. Some radiographers may not have witnessed trauma at such a scale, whether in terms of the seriousness of injuries or the sheer volume of patients attending. In some cases, such as terrorist attacks, relentless media coverage will impact on the ability to cope with emotions after the event, as they are constantly triggered. The planning should include emotional and psychological support for both during and after such an event. When undertaking mobile imaging on multiple patients, a systematic approach is essential, and an extra staff member will be invaluable. It is likely to be a hectic environment with lots of people carrying out their own roles. Staff may work within the Advanced Trauma Life Support (ATLS) protocol, which is a systemic approach to the identification of life-threatening injuries, and imaging will take place at a specific point within this protocol. It is important to identify the lead doctor and take instruction from them.

Advanced Trauma Life Support

ATLS is not limited to the major incident scenario, but is used on all victims of acute trauma. It standardises the multi-professional approach to patient management. The aim is to identify and treat the most significant injuries in a timely manner to reduce resuscitation times and minimise the risk of death. Death occurs in three peaks:

1. at the time of injury due to overwhelming injury to major organs;
2. several hours after injury because of hypoxia or haemorrhage, for example, causes that may be preventable if identified and treated quickly;
3. days or weeks after the injury due to sepsis or multiple organ failure, for example.

Trauma care is directed at the preventable deaths that occur within hours of the injury, and this is commonly referred to as the golden hour, comprising assessment and treatment at the scene of the accident, evaluation and treatment in the ED, and transfer to definitive care.

Good judgement is needed in pre-hospital care, and a decision around treating at the scene prior to transfer, or moving the patient with minimal input, for example management of airway or realignment of limbs, is vital in achieving a good outcome. Delays in transporting the patient can impact on the outcome.

Once the call is received from the ambulance service that a trauma patient is on route to the ED, a team, comprising clinical and ancillary staff, will be called to the emergency room. The clinical team will receive the patient and carry out a complete evaluation to identify any injuries and instigate a management plan. This team is led by the team lead, who is generally the most experienced member of staff present when the patient arrives. They will have a 'hands-off' approach, obtaining history from the paramedics, directing team members and having oversight of the assessment process. They will evaluate the information coming from each healthcare professional, prioritise investigations, receive results and formulate the management plan. They will have the final say on clinical decisions and discussions with relatives, and they will debrief staff at the end of the trauma call.

Throughout the period of care, the team lead will liaise with the scribe who documents all information as the clinical record of attendance. This is a clinical member of the team, and they will document such things as time of arrival and mechanism of injury. Physical findings such as vital signs and injuries will be documented, along with a record of investigation results, fluids or drugs administered and personnel present.

An anaesthetist will also be present. They are responsible for airway management, initiating intubation and ventilation as appropriate, and cervical spine control and, if surgical procedures are required, they will provide the anaesthesia. They will monitor vital signs, passing these to the team lead at regular intervals, and lead on fluid and drug administration.

Surgeons will also be present, with the general surgeon usually being responsible for the primary survey, comprising assessment of the head, thorax and abdomen. They may need to perform emergency surgery, such as thoracotomy or diagnostic peritoneal lavage. The orthopaedic surgeon will assess the spine, pelvis and limbs, apply emergency immobilisation devices and dress wounds. Other surgeons will be informed so that they can prepare to attend, if necessary, for example a neurosurgeon, plastic surgeon and thoracic surgeon. The anaesthetist and surgeons will be supported by an operating department practitioner and junior doctors and nursing staff from the ED.

Ancillary staff, such as porters, will act as runners, taking samples to the laboratories or going for equipment. Other staff will be present, such as a haematologist, a biochemist and a radiographer. The computed tomography (CT) scanning team, theatres and Intensive Care Unit will be informed so that they can start preparing for receipt of the patient. The whole team will work simultaneously, focusing on:

- A airway management and cervical spine control;
- B breathing and oxygenation;
- C circulation and bleeding;
- D disability;
- E environment and exposure.

The Role of the Radiographer

On receipt of the trauma call, the radiographer must gather all equipment and attend the emergency room prior to the patient arriving. They will also identify the team lead and take instruction from them. They will make sure those who need lead protection put it on before the patient arrives. It is important to follow local procedures for checking patient identity and pregnancy status and be ready to X-ray the patient when told to do so. This is generally within the primary survey, and X-rays must be performed in the order advised. Immediate life-threatening, but not obvious, injuries need excluding first. Always be ready to move yourself and the equipment away from the patient quickly if necessary.

Further imaging may be needed when the secondary survey is carried out. This will be after the patient has been resuscitated and stabilised and had a detailed head-to-toe clinical examination. It may involve multiple X-ray images, which, where possible, can be done within the department but may need to be done in the emergency room.

CHAPTER SUMMARY

- Managing multiple mobile X-ray examinations in a major incident requires good planning and communication with the ED team lead.
- In cases of major trauma, the team in the ED may follow the ATLS protocol for patient management.

REFERENCE

1. Civil Contingencies Act 2004 (Contingency Planning) Regulations 2005. Available at www.legislation.gov.uk/uksi/2005/2042/contents/made.

7. ADULT MOBILE RADIOGRAPHY TECHNIQUE

Radiographic technique in mobile X-ray imaging is relatively straight-forward, with challenges only being introduced dependent on the environment in which the patient is being nursed. By far the greatest number of mobile X-ray examinations performed are chest examinations. Predominantly, patients requiring a chest X-ray are imaged in an erect, supine, semi-erect or occasionally a decubitus position. It is better, when possible, to always image a patient in the erect position, as it is easier to position the patient, the breathing is better regulated and the patient can take a good breath in. This is helped by the gravitational pull of the abdominal organs ensuring that more of the lung fields can be seen. In addition, if there is a pleural effusion or any free fluid within the chest cavity, then this is better visualised with a horizontal beam.

It is not likely that a patient requiring a mobile X-ray chest image to be performed is well enough to achieve the postero-anterior (PA) position, so antero-posterior (AP) imaging is generally done. Occasionally a patient who is being barrier nursed, for example, may require a mobile chest X-ray and it may be possible to achieve this in a PA position. Additionally, if heart size assessment is an important factor for imaging, then a PA chest is recommended. Of course, if the patient is intubated then an erect image is probably not likely, but a semi-erect image may be possible. During the COVID-19 pandemic, patients were being nursed in the prone position to improve oxygen absorption in the lungs. Patients were imaged prone, as the efforts of turning a patient for an AP chest X-ray were immense.

The exposure should be done at maximum inspiration, and this may require the radiographer to watch for chest or abdomen movements if the patient is unresponsive and not able to follow commands to breathe in and hold their breath.

Mobile chest radiography can be performed for a number of reasons:

- to follow up known disease;
- to make a new diagnosis in the case of patient deterioration;
- to assess for position of:
    - an endotracheal tube;
    - a nasogastric tube;
    - a nasojejunal tube;
    - chest drains;
    - vascular catheters.

STANDARD STEPS FOR ALL PROCEDURES

- Identity and pregnancy checks, if appropriate, must be completed by the radiographer prior to imaging. If the patient is intubated or unresponsive, then checks must be made against the patient's wrist band.
- All attempts must be made to optimise imaging while minimising dose, and it is important to use collimation.
- All artefacts should be clear of the lung fields where possible.
- Depending on the patient's condition they may need immobilising or supporting to maintain position, which can be done by a staff member or by using pillows or radiolucent foam pads.
- Use detector covers to reduce the risk of cross infection or bodily fluids entering the detector.
- Often, working in pairs is easier (**Figure 7.1**). One radiographer can position the patient while the other concentrates on the imaging equipment. Additionally, there is somebody on hand who understands what you are trying to achieve if positioning is challenging.
- It is good practice to clean the machine before and after use.
- Annotate images, indicating patient position.

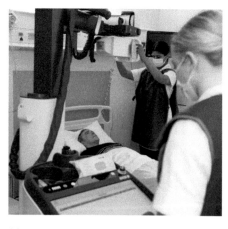

Figure 7.1 Working in pairs when doing mobile imaging.

CHEST IMAGING

The patient should be imaged in the erect position, when possible, for the reasons outlined previously. All exposures are taken on full inspiration, which can be achieved if the patient is able to respond to instruction or may require close visualisation of the chest and exposure to be initiated when the chest expands if the patient is unable to respond to instruction. Ensuring that the whole chest is included on the image can be difficult if the patient is of a large body habitus. Consider adjusting the detector from a portrait to a landscape position. In all cases the median sagittal plane should be in the middle of the detector and the upper edge of the detector should be level with the upper border of the shoulders. A useful suggestion is to include around 1 cm of detector above the upper border of the shoulders to allow for the slight raising of the shoulders during inspiration. Where possible, the focus-to-receptor distance (FRD) should be 180 cm. If supine, the maximum distance possible should be used.

Postero-anterior Erect Chest X-ray

If the patient can achieve the PA position, it is similar to that performed using static equipment. The patient is asked to sit with their legs over the side of the bed/trolley. A foam pad or pillow can be placed on their lap to support the detector so that it is in close contact with the front of the chest and the chin is resting on the top. It is important to make sure that the upper edge of the detector is above the patient's shoulder level and that the arms are rotated at the shoulders and extended around the detector.

Antero-posterior Erect Chest X-ray

If the patient is not stable in the PA position, the best AP projection is achieved when the patient is able to sit upright. Occasionally, a patient may not be stable if seated in an erect position, and a semi-erect or supine examination would be preferable in this instance.

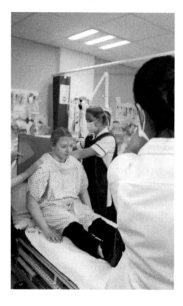

Figure 7.2 Positioning the patient and detector for an AP erect chest X-ray.

- The patient should be sitting upright in bed or on the trolley and the detector placed behind them (**Figure 7.2**).
- To stabilise the detector, it may be beneficial to place a pillow behind the patient with the detector between the patient and the pillow.
- The detector should be adjusted so that the upper border of the detector is visible above the shoulders. This will ensure that the apices are included on the image.
- Check that the lateral chest walls are also included within the detector field. If the patient is of large body habitus it may not be possible to see the detector behind the patient. Make sure that, when positioning the patient, the median sagittal plane is in the middle of the detector. Adjusting the detector from a portrait to a landscape position may be helpful.
- Make sure that the patient is not rotated and that the shoulders are equidistant from the detector.
- Rotate the arms internally to move the scapula from over the lung fields.

- Using an FRD of 180 cm, position the tube so that the horizontal central ray is perpendicular to the long axis of the sternum. This may require some caudal angulation if the patient is unable to sit perfectly upright.
- Centre to the level of T7, which can be found by identifying the sternal notch and centring 7–10 cm below this, or midway between the sternal notch and xiphisternum.

Supine Antero-posterior Chest X-ray

For those unable to sit up, a supine chest X-ray will need to be performed.

- The patient will be lying down in bed or on the trolley. The detector can be placed directly underneath them or, if they are on a trolley with an imaging tray, the detector can be placed in the tray (**Figure 7.3**). If there is no tray, then aids such as detector sliders should be used to minimise moving and handling.
- The detector should be positioned so that the upper border of the detector is visible above the shoulders. This will ensure that the apices are included on the image.
- Checking that the lateral chest walls are included involves standing at the top of the trolley and crouching down to see where the

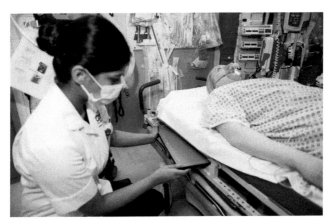

Figure 7.3 Positioning the detector in the tray underneath the trolley for a supine chest X-ray.

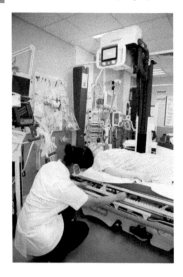

Figure 7.4 AP supine chest X-ray with the tube raised to the highest point to achieve the greatest FRD possible.

detector is placed in relation to the patient. Adjustments can be made to the position of the detector so that the median sagittal plane is in the middle of it.

■ Make sure that the patient is not rotated and that the shoulders are equidistant from the detector.

■ Rotate the arms internally to move the scapula from over the lung fields.

■ It will not be possible to raise the tube enough to achieve an FRD of 180 cm; so, use the maximum FRD possible (**Figure 7.4**), position the tube so that the vertical central ray is perpendicular to the long axis of the sternum.

■ Centre to the level of T7, which can be found by identifying the sternal notch and centring 7–10 cm below this, or midway between the sternal notch and xiphisternum.

Antero-posterior Semi-erect Chest X-ray

If the patient is unable to sit upright, in preference to doing a supine image, it may still be possible to achieve a partial erect image, referred to as a semi-erect chest X-ray. Sitting the patient up as much as possible, while maintaining safe practice, will still enable fluid levels to be

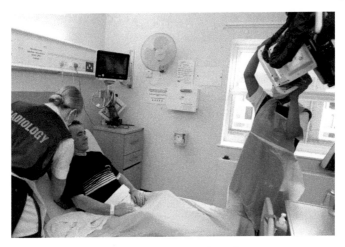

Figure 7.5 Patient positioned for a semi-erect chest X-ray.

seen on the image. Pillows and pads may be used to support the patient if they are not able to maintain the position themselves. The amount of inspiration may be reduced the closer the patient is to lying supine, as it is harder to take a deep breath when lying flat. The X-ray tube will need to be angled to reflect the angle on the detector, while still maintaining a central ray that is perpendicular to the long axis of the sternum (**Figure 7.5**).

Lateral Decubitus Chest X-ray

If the image is being performed to demonstrate fluid levels or pneumothorax, but the patient is unable to be positioned for an erect chest X-ray, then a lateral decubitus image may be performed. Both pleural effusions and free air can be difficult to see if the patient is imaged supine. Fluid will collect at the lowest point, which will be the back of the pleural cavity and air will rise to the highest point, which will be the front of the pleural cavity. Only to the experienced eye will the subtle signs associated with these be identified on the supine image.

A PA projection is preferred to minimise heart magnification; however, if the patient is unable to achieve this position, then an AP projection is acceptable if heart size assessment is not important.

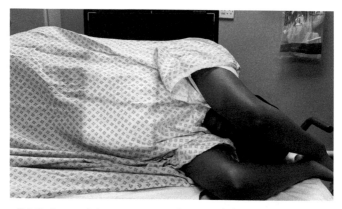

Figure 7.6 Patient and detector position for an AP left lateral decubitus chest X-ray.

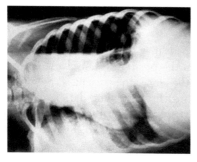

Figure 7.7 Lateral decubitus chest image demonstrating a pneumothorax and pleural effusion.

- The patient is turned onto their side (**Figure 7.6**).
    - If looking for fluid levels associated with a pleural effusion, the patient needs to lie on the affected side so that the fluid will collect at the lowest point within the pleural cavity.
    - If looking for free air associated with a pneumothorax, the patient needs to lie on the unaffected side so that air will rise to the highest point and be seen against the rib cage of the affected lung (**Figure 7.7**).
- It may be necessary to raise the patient clear of the mattress using radiolucent foam pads.

- The detector is placed in front of the patient, or behind if doing the image AP, and supported in a vertical position against the chest wall with the median sagittal plane perpendicular to the detector.
- The patient's arms must be raised above their head so that they do not obscure the chest.
- Using an FRD of 180 cm, the collimated horizontal beam is centred to the level of T7, which is 7–10 cm below the sternal notch, or midway between the sternal notch and xiphisternum.
- As the beam is being directed horizontally, care should be taken to move those in the immediate vicinity who are not required and to issue lead protection to those who are.

Dorsal Decubitus Chest X-ray

If the patient cannot lie on their side, then a dorsal decubitus image may be performed.

- The patient will remain supine, raised on pads if necessary, and the detector positioned against the affected side (**Figure 7.8**).
- The patient's arms are raised and their neck extended so that neither are superimposed on the chest.
- Centre to the level of T7.
- As a horizontal beam is being used, remove those people who do not need to be in the immediate vicinity and provide lead protection to those who are unable to move.

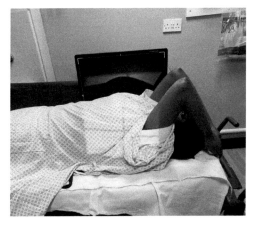

Figure 7.8 Patient and detector position for dorsal decubitus chest X-ray.

Essential Characteristics for Antero-posterior/ Postero-anterior Chest Images

The images should have the same characteristics as a PA chest obtained using static imaging equipment, whether obtained PA or AP, erect or supine (**Figure 7.9**).

- Six anterior or ten posterior ribs should be visible. It is likely that the supine image will demonstrate fewer anterior/posterior ribs if inspiration is affected by patient position.
- The lung fields should be clear of the scapulae.
- Clavicles should be equidistant from the spinous processes.
- The apices and the costophrenic angles should be clearly visible.

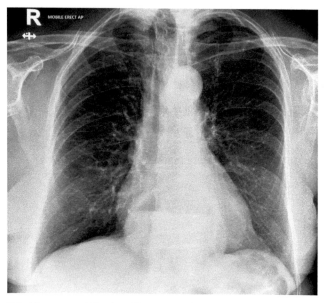

Figure 7.9 AP erect mobile chest X-ray; note the incarcerated hiatus hernia seen behind the heart shadow.

ABDOMINAL IMAGING

Abdominal imaging is not often performed outside the imaging department due to the complexities associated with achieving a diagnostic image. If imaging on a trolley, then an image comparable to one achieved on a patient trolley in the imaging department can be achieved. However, when imaging in a bed, due to the high exposure often required, a grid is generally needed and ensuring that the central ray is perpendicular to the grid is difficult. The risk of grid cut-off, where the grid strips absorb the primary ray, is high, leading to poor image quality. The advent of virtual grids has alleviated this problem as an algorithm in the equipment's software removes scattered radiation, but there are other challenges in mobile abdominal imaging. Placing the detector under the patient often requires several people to lift the patient, particularly if moving and handling devices such as detector slides are not available. Positioning the patient in relation to the detector is difficult, as often the abdomen is bigger than the detector and it is difficult to see if the patient is centralised.

A decision to request a mobile abdomen image will likely be made considering other imaging modalities available. If there is not an alternative to an abdomen X-ray, such as mobile ultrasound scanning, and/or the patient is too unstable to transfer to the imaging department, then a mobile X-ray image may be required to assess for free air, fluid levels or foreign bodies in, for example, a post-operative patient.

Erect abdominal imaging is rarely performed. Although some have identified value in the erect abdomen X-ray when assessing for small bowel obstruction,[1] this has perhaps been superseded by computed tomography (CT) scanning[2] and it is only carried out when access to CT is limited. If the clinical indication is suspected perforation, and the image is being obtained to assess for free air under the diaphragm, then this can be assessed on an erect chest image. The erect chest image has several benefits when assessing for acute abdomen pain. It allows for free air to be identified as the cause of pain, but also enables referred pain from a chest condition to be eliminated. In addition, the dose is much lower than that of an abdomen image. However, if the patient is unable to sit up for the erect chest X-ray, then decubitus imaging of the abdomen may be required. Free air will rise to the periphery of the abdomen when the patient lies on their side. Where possible, an FRD of 100 cm should be used.

Antero-posterior Supine Abdomen X-ray

- The patient lies supine and the detector (with or without a grid, depending on patient size and virtual grid availability) is placed in a portrait position either directly underneath the patient or in the imaging tray if the patient is being imaged on a trolley (**Figure 7.10**).
- The lower edge of the detector should be about 1 cm inferior to the symphysis pubis.
- The patient position is adjusted so that the median sagittal plane is perpendicular to the detector and, if possible, the lateral skin margins are within the detector parameters. It may be necessary to carry out two landscape images if it is not feasible to include all the abdomen on one image. Assess this prior to positioning the detector to minimise moving and handling.
- Centre in the midline at the level of the iliac crests, with an FRD of 100 cm.
- Expose on arrested expiration. If the patient is unable to follow instruction, then watch the chest and abdomen movements and expose when the patient breathes out.

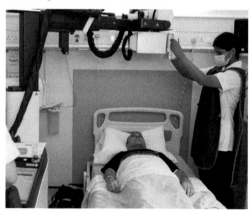

Figure 7.10 Position of patient and machine for supine abdomen X-ray.

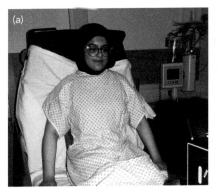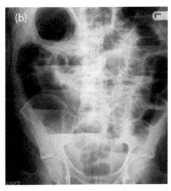

Figure 7.11 (a) Patient position for an erect abdomen X-ray; (b) AP erect abdomen image demonstrating small bowel obstruction, with gas in the bowel wall indicating imminent perforation.

Erect Abdomen X-ray

If access to CT scanning is not available, an erect abdomen X-ray may be required to look for fluid levels associated with small bowel obstruction (**Figure 7.11**).

- The patient should be supported to sit in an erect position similar to that of an erect chest X-ray, but their legs must be positioned so that the thighs do not superimpose the lower abdomen.
- The detector, with grid if being used, is placed in a portrait position behind the patient with the upper border of the detector placed 3 cm above the xiphisternum. This is usually controlled by the torso length of the patient and the detector may include much of the thorax in a smaller patient so good collimation is needed in this case.
- With an FRD of 100 cm, the horizontal beam is centred in the midline to the level of the iliac crests. If using a grid, make sure that the central ray is perpendicular to the detector and grid so that grid cut-off does not degrade the image.

Essential Characteristics for Abdomen Images

- There should be symmetry of the ribs and iliac crests to indicate no rotation of the patient (**Figure 7.12**).

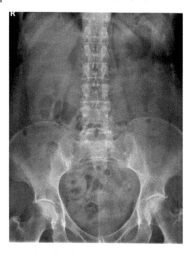

Figure 7.12 AP supine abdomen image demonstrating essential characteristics of the image. The diaphragms are not fully included, and discussion with the referrer will determine if another image across the upper abdomen is needed.

- The diaphragm should be included at the superior of the image.
- The symphysis pubis should be included on the inferior of the image.
- The soft tissues of the abdomen should be visible laterally; however, if the patient is of a large body habitus this may not be possible. It may be acceptable to include the bowel shadows only. Check with the referring clinician.

Lateral Decubitus Abdomen X-ray

If it is essential that the patient is assessed for free air, but they are unable to sit up for an erect chest image, then a decubitus image can be performed. The left lateral decubitus is preferred as free air will be easier to see as it outlines the liver.

- The patient should lie on their left side with their arms raised to prevent superimposition on the abdomen (**Figure 7.13**).
- The patient may need to be elevated on foam pads to raise the median sagittal plane to the middle of the detector so that the whole abdomen can be included. This is particularly important if a grid is being used.
- Do not position the detector in place at this point, as the patient should stay lying on their side for around 20 minutes before the exposure so that any free air can rise within the peritoneal cavity (**Figure 7.14**).

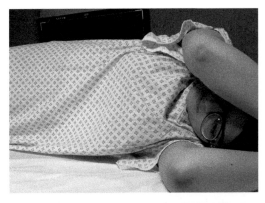

Figure 7.13 Patient and detector position for a lateral decubitus abdomen X-ray.

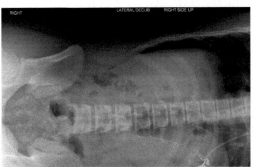

Figure 7.14 Left lateral decubitus image.

- If the patient is unable to lie on their left side, then a right lateral decubitus image can be performed.
- After 20 minutes, the detector, with or without a grid, should be stabilised vertically and in a portrait position against the patient, either anteriorly or posteriorly, with the lower border just inferior to the symphysis pubis.
- Using an FRD of 100 cm, the horizontal beam is centred in the midline at the level of the iliac crests with the central ray perpendicular to the detector.
- As a horizontal beam is being used, remove or protect other staff and patients in the immediate area.
- Exposure is taken on arrested expiration.
- Make sure that the image is marked correctly to indicate patient position.

Dorsal Decubitus Abdomen X-ray

If the patient is unable to lie on their side, then a dorsal decubitus abdomen image can be performed.

- The patient will remain supine and be elevated from the mattress by placing foam pads underneath them.
- The arms should be flexed with the hands placed above the head so that they do not obscure the abdomen (**Figure 7.15**).
- Like the lateral decubitus abdomen, the detector, with grid if being used, is stabilised vertically against the patient's side so that it is parallel to the median sagittal plane with the lower border just inferior to the symphysis pubis.
- Using an FRD of 100 cm, the horizontal central ray is centred to the lateral abdomen at the level of the iliac crests so that the anterior and posterior soft tissues are included. The central ray must be perpendicular to the detector.
- Remove or protect those in the immediate area.
- Exposure is taken on arrested expiration.

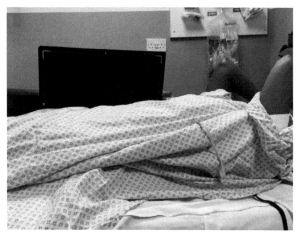

Figure 7.15 Positioning for a dorsal decubitus abdomen X-ray.

MUSCULOSKELETAL IMAGING

Although chest imaging is perhaps the most commonly performed of all mobile examinations, occasionally there will be a need to undertake imaging of the musculoskeletal system. An example of this is in a patient who has experienced major trauma when a trauma series is performed as part of the Advanced Trauma Life Support (ATLS) primary survey[3] as described in Chapter 6. The trauma series comprises an AP chest, AP pelvis and lateral cervical spine X-ray. The AP pelvis is carried out in the same manner as it would be in the imaging department, using the imaging tray underneath the trolley. The lateral cervical spine image will require a support for the mobile detector. Lateral cervical spine technique will be discussed.

Supine Lateral Cervical Spine X-ray

- The patient will be lying in the supine position and likely will have their neck supported in a head-immobilisation device.
- Position the mobile X-ray machine alongside the trolley so that a horizontal beam lateral image can be performed.
- Support the detector alongside the patient against the shoulder and parallel to the cervical spine (**Figure 7.16**).

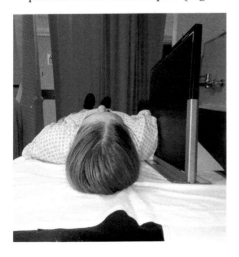

Figure 7.16 Support for detector alongside the patient for a lateral cervical spine X-ray.

97

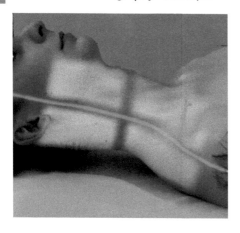

Figure 7.17 Centring at the level of C4 with the thyroid cartilage (Adam's apple) being the surface landmark.

- Using an FRD of 180 cm, centre the collimated beam to the level of C4, which can be found either 2.5 cm above the sternal notch or at the level of the thyroid cartilage (Adam's apple) (**Figure 7.17**).
- Remember to ask the patient to stretch their arms and reach down towards their feet. This will help to remove the shoulders from over the lower cervical spine. If they are unable to do this, and C7/T1 is not visible (**Figure 7.18a**), then ask one of the clinicians if they can grip the patient above the elbow and apply traction to the shoulders. Only a qualified professional should do this. Make sure that pregnancy checks are performed and lead protection is given to the clinician. Asking the patient to breathe out will also help to depress the shoulders.
- If C7/T1 is still not visualised, discuss with the lead clinician about doing a swimmer's projection (**Figure 7.18b**). In this projection, the arm closest to the detector is raised above the head and the arm furthest away is pulled downwards towards the feet. It is likely that the patient may be having a CT scan, so this projection is often not needed as they will obtain a CT of the cervical spine instead.

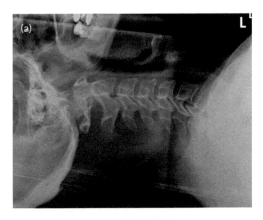

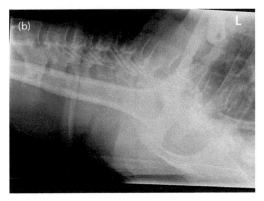

Figure 7.18 Lateral cervical spine images: (a) in head blocks with arm traction; (b) swimmer's projection.

Essential Characteristics for Lateral Cervical Spine Images

- The base of skull should be seen superiorly.
- The superior end plate of T1 should be seen inferiorly.
- The soft tissues should be seen anteriorly and posteriorly.
- The exposure should enable the soft tissues to be seen in detail anterior to the spine in order to exclude prevertebral soft tissue swelling.

99

CHAPTER SUMMARY

- When possible, an erect PA chest image is preferred, but if the patient is ill, it may be possible to do an AP erect image.
- Occasionally the patient requiring an X-ray may need to be imaged in the supine or, rarely, the prone position.
- Mobile abdomen imaging is not often performed, but when it is, care needs to be taken when using a grid to make sure that grid cut-off does not degrade the image.
- When performing decubitus imaging, be aware that a horizontal beam will be used, and this will require consideration of radiation protection for those in the vicinity.

REFERENCES

1. Lappas, J.C., Reyes, B.L. and Maglinte, D.D. Abdomen radiography findings in small-bowel obstruction: relevance to triage for additional diagnostic imaging. *American Journal of Roentgenology* 2001;**176**:167–174.
2. Amara, Y., Leppaniemi, A., Catena, F., Ansaloni, L., Sugrue, M., Fraga, G.P. et al. Diagnosis and management of small bowel obstruction in virgin abdomen: a WSES position paper. *World Journal of Emergency Surgery* 2021;**16**:article no. 36.
3. Thippeswamy, P.B. and Rajasekaran, R.B. Imaging in polytrauma – principles and current concepts. *Journal of Clinical Orthopaedics and Trauma* 2021;**16**:106–113.

8. PAEDIATRIC MOBILE RADIOGRAPHY TECHNIQUE

Radiographer training traditionally focuses on adult imaging; however, it is likely that imaging children will be a requirement of the radiographer's role as well. Throughout this chapter, the term 'child' will be used in reference to children of all ages and encompassing neonates (under the age of 28 days), infants (under the age of 1 year) and toddlers (under the age of 4 years). Although the theory of mobile imaging is the same as in adult imaging, the practicalities are often quite different. As discussed previously, mobile imaging should only be carried out on those whose clinical condition makes it unsafe for them to attend the imaging department and this is the same for children.

The differences, both physically and developmentally, between a pre-term neonate and an adolescent child pose a variety of challenges. Apart from the practical technique in achieving these images, there are also challenges to obtaining images of a good diagnostic quality, as bone mineralisation usually occurs in the third trimester, and normal bone density will not be present in the pre-term child (**Figure 8.1a**) when compared with an older child (**Figure 8.1b**). This can cause

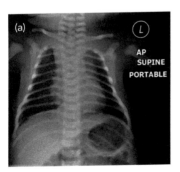
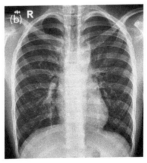

Figure 8.1 Antero-posterior (AP) chest images in (a) a neonate; (b) a 15-year-old child.

difficulties when using newer imaging technologies that utilise generic background-processing algorithms to enhance images.

Another key consideration when imaging children is radiation dose. It is well documented that a child's organs are more radio-sensitive than an adult's.[1] When justifying a request for a mobile examination, the type of examination and the resultant dose should always be considered using a benefit/risk analysis as outlined in Chapter 3. An example of this is when a clinician requests a chest and abdomen X-ray to assess for perforation. If the child is considered at risk of perforation, a mobile erect chest X-ray or, in exceptional circumstances, a lateral decubitus X-ray could be offered in the first instance. The results of this would enable the clinicians to decide if they should proceed with a mobile abdomen X-ray or whether it could potentially be carried out in the imaging department where optimum image quality and radiation dose can be better achieved.

While there may be challenges in dealing with older children when undertaking mobile imaging, the technique is very similar to that of adults. This chapter will concentrate on mobile radiography of neonates and very young children.

STANDARD STEPS FOR ALL PROCEDURES

- Identity and pregnancy checks, if appropriate, must be completed by the radiographer prior to imaging. Identity checks with the child can be difficult. Checks can be made with the carer, or against their name band. Extra care is needed in neonatal intensive care settings, as there are often multiple birth siblings with the same family name and normally the same date of birth, often making the only unique identifier the hospital number.
- Consent for imaging must be sought from the carer. The referrer or nurse in charge may have asked for consent if the carer is not likely to be present at the time of imaging.
- Make sure all those required to be present are wearing lead protection.
- All attempts must be made to optimise imaging while minimising radiation dose, and it is important to use appropriate collimation.
- All artefacts should be clear of the lung fields where possible; this is especially important in the pre-term, as sometimes the electrocardiogram (ECG) dots or a temperature probe can obscure

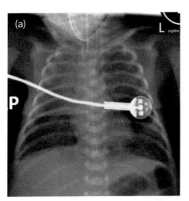 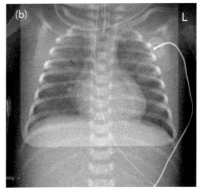

Figure 8.2 AP supine chest images demonstrating artefacts caused by (a) the temperature probe obscuring the left lung; (b) the ventilator circuit support device.

a complete lobe (**Figure 8.2a**). In addition, when imaging in the incubator tray, artefacts can be caused by structures between the child and the detector. **Figure 8.2b** demonstrates a rectangular area of increased density which is caused by the device used to support the ventilator circuit. This is tucked between the base of the incubator and the patient mattress and should be moved if using the tray.

- Depending on the child's age and condition they may need immobilising by a staff member or parent/carer. Ensure the patient holder is not pregnant and that records are completed. Clear instructions with a 'dry run' will ensure that the person holding the patient understands their responsibilities.

- Use detector covers to reduce the risk of cross infection or bodily fluids entering the detector (**Figure 8.3**).

- Place the anatomical marker in the field of view.

- When possible, all chest images must be taken on inspiration, whereas abdomen images are taken on expiration. In young children this may require a good view of the abdomen, as chest movement is often very subtle and the abdomen provides a clearer indication of the phase of respiration.

- It is good practice to clean the machine before and after use.

- Annotate the images indicating the position that the child was imaged in and the time of imaging, if there is no electronic time stamp.

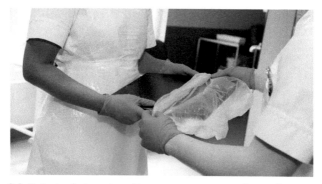

Figure 8.3 Detector being placed in a cover to protect it from infection and/or bodily fluids when imaging children.

CHEST IMAGING

Whenever practical, an erect chest examination would be preferable; however, in paediatric imaging this is not always possible due to the age of the child. Erect radiography of the chest should not be performed unless the child is developmentally of an age where they naturally are trying to sit upright and have some level of head control. When mobile radiography is requested, this is normally because the child is too unwell to attend the department. This alone would indicate that they are not able to sit up.

When imaging in a Neonatal Intensive Care Unit (NICU) or Special Care Baby Unit (SCBU), most incubators have an inbuilt detector tray (**Figure 8.4**). These are designed for the radiographer to place the detector in, so it is beneath the patient. Some units routinely use these trays whereas others reserve their use for only the most unwell children. If the child is at risk of sudden reduction in temperature, then they will be nursed through ports in the incubator and the tray is likely to be used. Use of the incubator tray for imaging must be discussed locally. See Chapter 5 for more information on use of the tray.

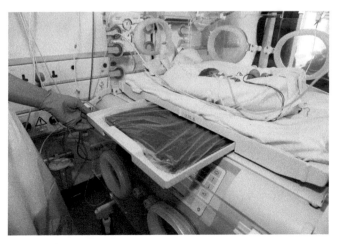

Figure 8.4 Incubator tray in use.

Antero-posterior Supine Chest X-ray (under 6 months of age)

- If the baby is in an incubator, the detector may or may not be in the incubator tray.
- The child should be placed flat on their back with the upper edge of the detector level with the superior borders of the shoulders. The nurse looking after them must place the head and pelvis in a neutral position with the median sagittal plane adjusted so that it is at right angles to the middle of the detector (**Figure 8.5**). A 15° wedge pad may be used under the upper body to enable the sternum to be perpendicular to the central ray (**Figure 8.6a**). This angle may also be achieved by leaving the head end of the bed/incubator slightly elevated (**Figure 8.6b**).
- The focus-to-receptor (FRD) distance should be 110 cm.
- The collimated vertical beam should be centred midway between the sternal notch and the xiphisternum, at the level of the intermammillary line.

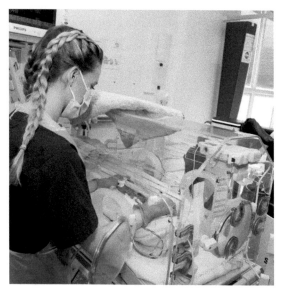

Figure 8.5 Positioning the baby with head and pelvis in a neutral position.

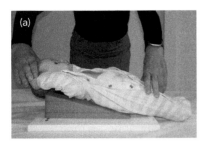 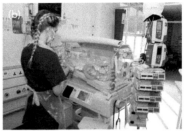

Figure 8.6 Angulation applied by (a) use of foam pad; (b) tilt of incubator.

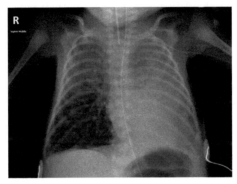

Figure 8.7 AP chest image performed with arms abducted at the side of the body to demonstrate line position.

- If imaging is to look at the lung fields, a neonate or baby can be immobilised by raising their flexed arms slightly forward above their head to minimise scapulae superimposition on the lung fields (Figure 8.6a). However, for line positioning, arms should be in a neutral position and slightly abducted at the side of the body to obtain best accuracy of the line position (**Figure 8.7**).[2]

Erect Chest X-ray (over 6 months of age)

- The child sits supported with their back against the detector, with the upper edge of the detector level with the superior borders of the shoulders. The head should be in a neutral position.
- While developmentally it is recognised that a child should have some head control and be able to sit upright with some assistance

107

by 6 months, this will vary from child to child and the radiographer should assess the situation once they are at the child's bedside.

- If the child is being nursed in a cot, drop one of the cot sides as low as it can go, seat the child against the other cot side and place the detector between the cot side and the child. The median sagittal plane must be adjusted so that it is at right angles to the middle of the detector.

- If the child is being nursed in a bed but can sit up for their imaging, the bed position should be adjusted to an upright or seated position (head up, feet lowered) and the child then positioned in an erect position, with the detector placed behind their back. This is not dissimilar to the technique for the AP erect chest examination in adults.

- With an FRD of 180 cm, the collimated horizontal beam is angled caudally so that the central ray is at right angles to the sternum and centred midway between the sternal notch and the xiphisternum.

- Immobilisation may be required, and this could simply be the use of pillows or foam pads (or cuddly toys) to provide additional support.

Prone Chest X-ray

Occasionally a child is being nursed prone and it may be possible to image them prone, thus minimising handling. Discuss this with the clinical team to determine what is in the child's best interest.

- Place the detector under the anterior aspect of their chest, with the upper edge of the detector level with the superior borders of the shoulders.

- The median sagittal plane should be adjusted to ensure that it is at right angles to the middle of the detector. Head rotation should be minimised. In neonates it is often useful to insert a small roll under their hips to help minimise rotation.

- With an FRD of 110 cm, the collimated vertical beam is angled so that the central ray is perpendicular to the detector and centred midway between T3 and T4.

Lateral or Dorsal Decubitus Chest X-ray

If the image is required to demonstrate fluid levels or pneumothorax, but the child is unable to be positioned for an erect chest X-ray, then a decubitus image may be performed. These can be useful in identifying a small effusion or pneumothorax. The child may need raising on foam pads.

- For a lateral decubitus image, the child lies on their side. If looking for fluid levels they need to lie on the affected side, and if looking for free air they need to lie on the unaffected side. The detector is positioned behind the child and the median sagittal plane adjusted to be at right angles to the detector.
- It may not be possible to lie a child on their side, especially neonates, so a dorsal decubitus image will be needed. The child remains supine and the detector is positioned at the side of the child with the upper edge of the detector level with the superior border of the shoulders. The median sagittal plane should be adjusted to ensure that it is parallel to the detector. This technique produces a lateral chest X-ray.
- In both positions, care should be taken to support the head in a neutral position. Arms should be placed above the head.
- The detector and child may need support to achieve and maintain these positions.
- With an FRD of 110 cm, the collimated horizontal beam is at right angles to the detector and the centring point is at the level of the intermammillary line. As the beam is being directed horizontally (**Figure 8.8**), care needs to be given to those in the immediate vicinity, and not required to be there, to ensure that they can

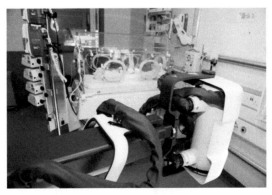

Figure 8.8 Position of X-ray tube for decubitus imaging.

vacate the designated controlled area while the exposure is being undertaken.

Essential Characteristics for Antero-posterior Chest Images

- If performed at peak inspiration, full lung fields should be clearly visualised to include apices, costophrenic angles and rib edges laterally (**Figure 8.9**). Six anterior or nine to ten posterior ribs should be visible above the right costophrenic angle.
- The area to include is from C3 superiorly to L1 inferiorly and the soft tissue margins laterally. This should be no more than 1 cm lateral to the widest point of the chest.
- Scapulae should be clear of the lung fields if possible and the clavicles should be equidistant from the manubrium.
- The image should be clear of all artefacts where possible, including temperature probes and ECG leads crossing the body (**Figure 8.10**). This is especially important in the pre-term, as sometimes the ECG dots themselves can obscure a complete lobe.
- Make sure that the image is annotated.

If the image is not diagnostically acceptable, then it is important to recognise how to correct any errors. **Figure 8.11a** demonstrates a rotated chest image. This error is creating the false impression of a pneumothorax. On the periphery of the image, it is possible to see the chin is turned to the left, so the head position has not been neutralised prior to

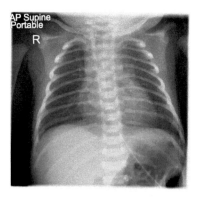

Figure 8.9 AP supine neonatal chest image demonstrating relevant anatomy.

exposure. The body has been allowed to rotate to the left, seen by elongation of the left ribs. This can be corrected by neutralising the head and pelvis and using foam pads to maintain this position. **Figure 8.11b** demonstrates a chest image that is lordotic indicating that the head was not elevated either using a foam pad under the detector or by raising the head end of the incubator. There is also slight rotation to the left, demonstrated by elongation of the left ribs.

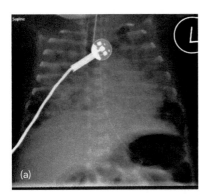 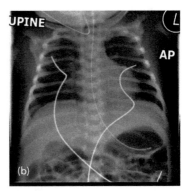

Figure 8.10 Supine AP neonatal chest images demonstrating (a) temperature probe overlying the endotracheal tube; (b) ECG leads over the lung fields.

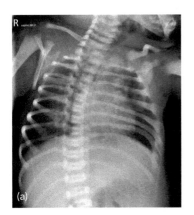 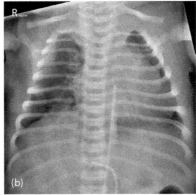

Figure 8.11 AP supine chest images demonstrating (a) rotation to the left; (b) lordosis.

ABDOMINAL IMAGING

Abdominal imaging is not very common in children as ultrasound is generally performed. However, it is often performed in a NICU or SCBU setting to look for suspected gastrointestinal (GI) obstruction or necrotising enterocolitis (NEC). Although NEC is a clinical emergency in which the bowel tissue starts to die due to infection and inflammation,[3] GI obstruction is the most common surgical emergency in a neonate, often caused by intestinal atresia, Hirschsprung disease, malrotation or meconium ileus.[4] Both NEC and GI obstruction require a supine abdomen X-ray as the first line of investigation.

Mobile decubitus imaging is carried out to look for free intra-peritoneal air in the abdomen. It is not carried out routinely but may be required if the child is acutely unwell and erect chest imaging or computed tomography (CT) scan cannot be performed. The ideal position is the left lateral decubitus; however, if this cannot be achieved, a dorsal decubitus is acceptable. As with decubitus chest imaging (**Figure 8.8**), as the beam is being directed horizontally, care needs to taken to ensure those in the vicinity and not required to be there can vacate the designated controlled area while the exposure is being undertaken.

Supine Antero-posterior Abdomen X-ray

- If the baby is in an incubator, the detector may or may not be in the incubator tray (**Figure 8.12a**).
- The child lies supine. To ensure no rotation, the hips should be neutral with the legs in extension, and the median sagittal plane adjusted at right angles to the middle of the detector.
- With an FRD of 100 cm, the collimated vertical beam is at right angles to the detector and centred between the xiphisternum and inferior pubic rami (**Figure 8.12b**).
- Place anatomical marker in the field of view.

Lateral or Dorsal Decubitus Abdomen X-ray

If it is essential that the child is assessed for free air, but if they are unable to sit up for an erect chest image, then a decubitus image can

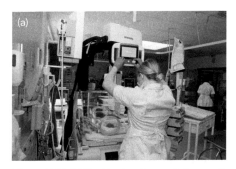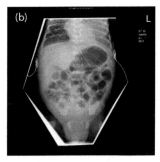

Figure 8.12 (a) Positioning for an abdomen X-ray in an incubator; (b) resultant image of the abdomen demonstrating a nasogastric tube in the stomach.

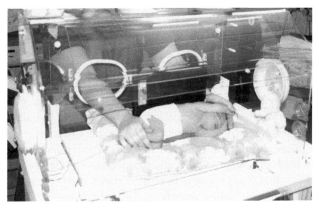

Figure 8.13 Detector and patient position for left lateral decubitus abdomen X-ray.

be performed. The left lateral decubitus is preferred as free air will rise and outline the liver. If the child is too unstable to lie on their side, a dorsal decubitus image may be performed. The child may need raising on foam pads.

- For the left lateral decubitus image (**Figure 8.13**), the child is turned on to their left side with their back against the detector. The median sagittal plane is adjusted to be at right angles to the detector.

113

- For the dorsal decubitus image, the child is supine, and the detector is supported adjacent to the side of the child. The median sagittal plane is adjusted to be parallel to the detector. A lateral abdomen image is achieved.
- The collimated horizontal beam is centred midway between the xiphisternum and the inferior pubic rami using an FRD of 100 cm.
- Care should be taken to support the head in a neutral position. Arms should be placed above the head.
- As a horizontal beam is being used, make sure that those in the vicinity are moved or adequately protected.
- Place anatomical marker in the field of view.

Essential Image Characteristics for Supine and Lateral Decubitus Abdomen Images

- The area to be included is from the diaphragm superiorly to the inferior pubic rami inferiorly, and the soft tissue margins laterally (**Figure 8.14a**). It is also important to include the inguinal area in males if the clinical information relates to this area.
- When imaging in the lateral decubitus position, flexion of the hips may result in the inferior abdomen not being easily visualised. This can be corrected by extending the legs during exposure.
- The image should be clear of all artefacts where possible, including ECG leads crossing the body and temperature probes overlying the liver. If it is not possible to remove them, turn them so that the leads are positioned away from the body. Take care with any blankets that the child may be lying on. **Figure 8.14b** demonstrates an abdomen image with multiple areas of lucency caused by a neonatal cooling blanket used to treat hypoxia. Failure to recognise this may result in a misdiagnosis. Identifying that the cooling blanket may cause artefacts and seeking guidance on removing it prior to imaging will minimise this risk.
- Make sure that the image is annotated.

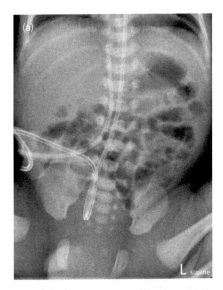

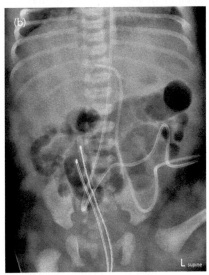

Figure 8.14 AP supine neonatal abdomen image (a) demonstrating essential characteristics; (b) demonstrating blanket artefacts.

CHEST AND ABDOMEN IMAGING

Imaging of the chest and abdomen in one single exposure is not technic-ally possible in the adult environment, and in most paediatric environ-ments would be considered poor radiographic practice. However, when performing mobile paediatric radiography there can be occasions where imaging of the chest and abdomen as one whole image is acceptable. Those instances are limited and often occur in the acute settings of neo-natal/paediatric intensive care or paediatric high-dependency setting. Imaging can be justified to look for placement of an umbilical arterial catheter, umbilical venous catheter, peripherally inserted venous lines (often called long lines), or nasogastric, nasojejunal or trans-anasto-motic nasogastric tubes.

Supine Chest and Abdomen X-ray (<6 months)

■ If the baby is in an incubator, the detector may or may not be in the incubator tray.

■ The child lies supine with the upper edge of the detector level with the superior borders of the shoulders.

■ The head and pelvis should be in a neutral position and the median sagittal plane is adjusted at right angles to the middle of the detector.

■ As imaging is often required for line position, studies have shown that they should be taken with the arms in a neutral position by the side of the body to obtain best accuracy of the line position.

■ A 15° pad may be used under the child's upper body to facilitate the alignment of the sternum to the X-ray beam at right angles (Figure 8.6a). This may also be achieved by leaving the head end of the bed/incubator slightly elevated (Figure 8.6b).

■ With an FRD of 100 cm, the collimated vertical beam is angled until it is at right angles to the sternum and centred in the midline at the level of the inferior ribs, which can be found between the xiphisternum and the iliac crest (**Figure 8.15**).

■ Place anatomical marker in the field of view.

■ The exposure is taken on full inspiration when possible.

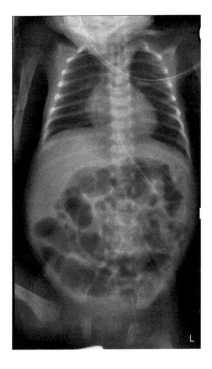

Figure 8.15 Chest and abdomen image obtained in one exposure.

Essential Image Characteristics for a Chest and Abdomen Image

- Characteristics of both chest and abdomen imaging should be aimed for.
- The exposure should be performed at peak inspiration enabling full lung fields to be clearly visualised.
- The areas to be included should be superiorly to C3, inferiorly to the inferior pubic rami and laterally to the soft tissue margins. It is also important to include the inguinal area in males if the clinical information relates to this area.
- Clavicles should be equidistant from the manubrium with six anterior or nine/ten posterior ribs visible above the right costophrenic angle.
- All artefacts should be clear of the chest and abdomen.
- Make sure that the image is annotated.

CHAPTER SUMMARY

- Children vary in size, from the pre-term neonate to the adult-size adolescent, and present different challenges when undertaking mobile examinations.
- A parent or carer may be needed to provide patient assistance. Make sure that pregnancy checks are done, when appropriate, and lead protection is provided.
- Communication skills and the reliance on observational skills to ascertain the optimum time to take the image are essential.
- Remove all artefacts from the field of view if possible, as they can obscure important anatomy in a very small neonate.

REFERENCES

1. Care Quality Commission. Findings from CQC's IR(ME)R Inspection Programme of Specialist Paediatric Radiologist Services. Available at www.cqc.org.uk/sites/default/files/20190708_irmer_paediatric_radiology_inspection_programme_report.pdf
2. Fridolfsson, P.E.J. Ultrasound-guided peripherally inserted central catheter placement in extremely low birth weight neonates. *Neonatal Network* 2022;**41**(1):21–37.
3. Soni, R., Katana, A., Curry, J.I., Humphries, P. and Huertas-Ceballos, A. How to use abdominal X-rays in preterm infants suspected of developing necrotising enterocolitis. *Archives of Disease in Childhood – Education and Practice* 2020;**105**:50–57.
4. Afzali, N., Malek, A. and Abasi, N. Comparison of abdominal X-ray findings and results of surgery in neonates with gastrointestinal obstruction. *International Journal of Pediatrics* 2019;**7**(1):8877–8880.

SECTION 3
THEATRE RADIOGRAPHY

9. SURGICAL SPECIALTIES REQUIRING FLUOROSCOPIC IMAGING

Theatre fluoroscopy can be undertaken for elective and acute surgical procedures and is required by numerous specialties to guide surgical interventions. Understanding the specialty will help the radiographer prepare for the procedure being performed. Regardless of the specialty, there is normally a large team of staff and the radiographer needs to quickly embed themselves within that team. Communication is key to achieving a safe and successful outcome to the procedure, especially when acquisition of good diagnostic images is dependent on patient position in relation to the imaging equipment. Communication is discussed in more detail in Chapter 1, Introduction to Mobile Imaging.

In addition, there will be a lot of equipment, much of which is sterile and must not be touched (**Figure 9.1**). This may include an anaesthetic machine if the patient is having a general anaesthetic, suction machines and sterile trolleys of equipment associated with the surgical procedure. There may also be specialised equipment for some procedures, such as a Hemosep, a blood transfusion machine used in major surgical procedures, or a surgical microscope for carrying out microsurgery. Additionally, the mobile fluoroscopy machine is a specialised piece of equipment, and it may require draping to ensure sterility is maintained.

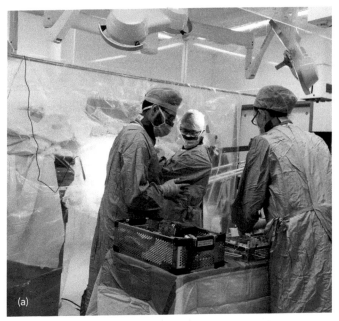

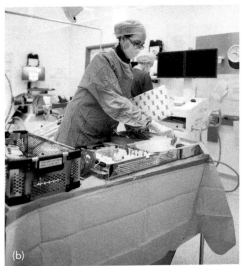

Figure 9.1 Surgical teams and equipment in an operating theatre.

ORTHOPAEDIC SURGERY

Orthopaedic surgery using mobile fluoroscopy guidance commonly occurs following trauma to support the surgeon in treating injuries involving the musculoskeletal system. There are some generic procedures that are used for numerous different body parts. Manipulation under anaesthetic (MUA) is used if a fracture is likely to be stable once the correct anatomical position has been achieved (**Figure 9.2a**). It simply involves the surgeon manipulating the fracture into normal alignment and does not involve any surgical metalwork being inserted into the fracture site. MUA can be performed on all limbs of the appendicular skeleton and is usually performed in the theatre environment if an attempt at manipulation has been unsuccessful in the Emergency Department or in the ward setting. MUA is less invasive than open reduction with internal fixation (ORIF) and it has reduced infection rates, has shorter anaesthetic time and is less traumatic for the patient. MUA is often the first option for a dislocated joint for the same reasons. ORIF is performed if a fracture is complex and unlikely to be stable following MUA (**Figure 9.2b**). Metalwork, in the form of wires, screws

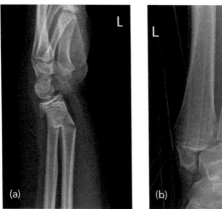
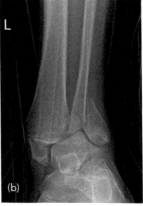

Figure 9.2 (a) Lateral wrist image demonstrating a stable injury suitable for MUA; (b) antero-posterior (AP) ankle image demonstrating an unstable injury requiring ORIF.

or pins, for example, is used to stabilise the fracture (**Figure 9.3**). In addition to being used to stabilise appendicular fractures, ORIF can also be performed on the axial skeleton.

There are also some procedures that are relevant only to a single body part, such as a dynamic hip screw for fractures of the femoral neck and a proximal humeral internal locking system procedure for shoulder surgery. Due to the nature of orthopaedic trauma and the associated complexity of the injuries, the various techniques often must be adapted.

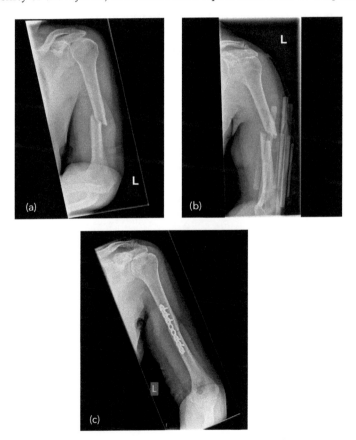

Figure 9.3 AP humerus images demonstrating (a) a displaced fracture; (b) fracture position following manipulation and application of brace; (c) fracture position following ORIF due to instability at the fracture site.

NEUROSURGERY

Neurosurgery focuses on the treatment of conditions affecting the nervous system, that is, the brain and spinal cord. Radiographers are likely to be called upon to support the surgeon with fluoroscopic guidance in procedures such as microdiscectomy, laminectomy and posterior lumbar interbody fusion. In addition, radiographers will be required to support in pain clinics that undertake pain management procedures such as a trigeminal nerve block, facet joint injection and nerve root injection with or without a nerve block.

UROLOGY

Urology is a surgical subspeciality covering the diagnosis and treatment of disorders of the urinary tract from the kidneys to the urethra (**Figure 9.4**) and male reproductive organs. A common procedure is the insertion of stents, that is, small plastic tubes, into a ureter that has become blocked by, for example, a small kidney stone or a stricture from disease. The stent allows urine to flow freely between the kidney and the bladder. Other procedures, such as percutaneous nephrolithotomy and drain insertion, are also performed in urology theatres.

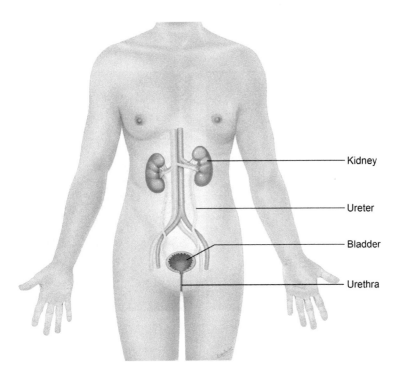

— Kidney

— Ureter

— Bladder

— Urethra

Figure 9.4 The urinary tract.

VASCULAR IMAGING

Vascular surgery often requires radiological visualisation of the blood vessels but does not usually include the vessels of the heart as this is generally classified as cardiac surgery. There are many methods of imaging the blood vessels including computed tomography (CT) and magnetic resonance imaging (MRI) (**Figure 9.5**). Although CT and MRI are less invasive, these techniques are not possible in a theatre environment and traditional angiography will be needed. Dynamic imaging will allow the surgeon to see the flow of contrast medium as it is injected into the vessels. If a vessel is narrowed, an angioplasty may be carried out at the same time. This involves insertion of a balloon catheter, which is inflated at the site of the narrowed vessel.

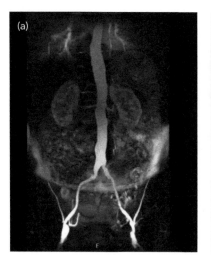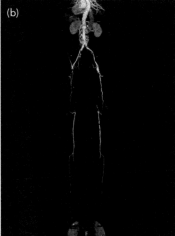

Figure 9.5 Vascular imaging using (a) a magnetic resonance scan and (b) a CT scan.

CARDIAC PACING

Cardiac angiography enables the heart and associated vessels to be visualised for diagnostic or treatment purposes and is often carried out in a static dedicated cardiac catheterisation suite. However, some procedures may be performed in a theatre setting with a vascular-enabled mobile fluoroscopy machine. This may be the case in a district general hospital when pacemaker insertion procedures are being performed without a dedicated imaging suite. This practice has been carried out for more than two decades following approval by the British Cardiovascular Society.[1] Cardiac pacing, also called cardiac rhythm management, is performed to treat bradycardia, a slow heart rate, by delivering an electrical stimulus to the chambers of the heart (**Figure 9.6**) when needed to manage the heart rhythm. The pacing rate is usually set to pace 'on demand' when the heart rate falls below 50 beats per minute. It is usually performed under local anaesthetic with conscious sedation.

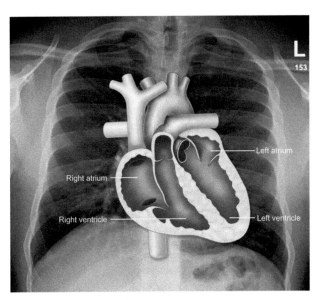

Figure 9.6 Chest image demonstrating the position of the heart chambers.

GENERAL SURGERY

General surgery encompasses a wide range of procedures from planned to surgical emergencies. The most common procedures in which mobile fluoroscopy is used are endoscopic retrograde cholangiopancreatography (ERCP) and cholangiography. Like cardiac pacing surgery, ERCP is often carried out in a static fluoroscopy suite; however, it can occasionally take place in theatre.

BRACHYTHERAPY

Brachytherapy is a form of radiotherapy in which seeds or small tubes containing a radiation source are placed into or close to a tumour to destroy cancerous cells. Fluoroscopy may be required during placement of the radiation source, most commonly for treatment of prostate cancer.

CHAPTER SUMMARY

- Theatre fluoroscopy is required by numerous specialties to support surgery.
- Understanding the surgical specialty will help to prepare the radiographer for the procedure being performed.
- Communication is key to achieving a safe and successful outcome to the procedure.

REFERENCE

1.   Leong, K.M., Pollard, C. and Cooke, C.J. Cardiology registrars and permanent pacemaker complication rates in a district general hospital – safety and service implications. *Clinical Medicine* 2014;**14**(1):34–37.

10. FLUOROSCOPY TECHNIQUE IN THEATRE

The aim of this chapter is to give the radiographer an understanding of the different types of theatre examinations and the technique required to obtain diagnostic images to assist with surgery.

The rationale behind imaging in theatre is generally easy to see, but theatre fluoroscopy can be seen as challenging, in particular by newly qualified radiographers when asked to attend theatre for the first time alone or by experienced radiographers who are attending theatre for a procedure with which they are unfamiliar.[1] It is essential that the radiographer understands their role in this environment, as they are an essential part of the team. Clearly they must be competent in the use of the mobile fluoroscopy machine, which may use an image intensifier or a flat plate detector for image acquisition (more detail on the differences between these two types of mobile fluoroscopy machine can be found in Chapter 2). In addition, they must also demonstrate other skills that will assist in alleviating the fear that is often experienced. Key skills and knowledge required include:

- preparing appropriately for the procedure;
- understanding the function and limitations of the imaging equipment to achieve high-quality diagnostic images to support the surgeon;
- communicating and demonstrating effective teamwork;
- knowledge of infection prevention and control and the ability to maintain a sterile environment;
- expertise in radiation safety and protection of all staff and the patient.

In addition to developing these skills, there is a lot to remember for each procedure. Chapter 4 presents a high-level workflow, but the specific imaging aspects of each procedure will be different. There are steps that are standard across all procedures, and these will be discussed before looking at each procedure and associated specific imaging requirements in detail.

Throughout this chapter it will be presumed that images are being acquired using a flat plate detector, the positioning of which will be explained for each procedure. If an intensifier is being used, it will still be placed in the same location for image acquisition.

STANDARD STEPS FOR ALL PROCEDURES

Safety Checks

- Identity and pregnancy checks, if appropriate, must be completed by the radiographer prior to the patient being anaesthetised, if possible. If the patient is already anaesthetised, local procedures should be followed, such as carrying out these checks with the anaesthetist or surgeon or checking the name band of the patient.
- Position the mobile fluoroscopy machine as indicated by the theatre staff. This will depend upon the surgery site and the position of the surgeon, but it is usual to be at 90° to the patient and on the opposite side to the surgeon. It is wise to check with the surgeon prior to the procedure commencing.
- Consider where the mobile fluoroscopy machine is plugged in. It is best not to have the cables crossing the floor of the theatre, as they can be a trip hazard.
- It is best practice to have the detector at the top (**Figure 10.1a**); however, this needs to be balanced against the fact that there is likely to be a very large air gap, resulting in increased skin dose to the patient, increased magnification, increased scatter and reduced image quality.
- The surgeon may prefer the detector to be underneath the table (**Figure 10.1b**) so that they have as much space to operate as possible and are not restricted by the detector position. The detector should be raised so that it is as close to the patient as possible. This also allows better use of the laser lights for positioning as they are generally found on the X-ray tube head. Depending on X-ray tube position, images may be acquired in the antero-posterior (AP) or postero-anterior (PA) positions and this is reflected throughout the chapter by indicating AP/PA for technique.

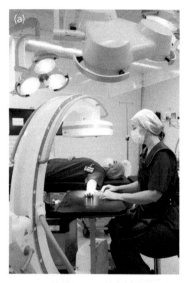

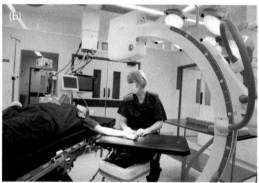

Figure 10.1 Detector position (a) at the top or above the patient and (b) at the bottom or below the patient.

Dose and Image Optimisation

- All attempts must be made to optimise imaging while minimising radiation dose.
- Be aware of staff who may not be wearing lead protection, including those who are scrubbed up and in sterile garments.

- It is important to use collimation to improve image quality, reduce radiation dose and scatter, and avoid imaging the surgeon's fingers. The iris collimator can generally be used, but occasionally lateral collimators may be required if available, when visualisation of the whole bone/limb is needed.
- Fluoroscopy must only be initiated on the request of the surgeon.
- If a laser light is available on the equipment, this will assist in ensuring the area of interest is in the middle of the field of view to maximise image quality and reduce radiation dose. It is particularly useful in the paediatric setting due to the size of the body part being imaged. Imaging on the periphery of the field of view will result in the collimators having to remain open, subsequently increasing radiation dose and reducing image quality. Use of a laser light can help more accurate centring prior to exposure.
- Images must be transferred to the reference screen between AP/PA and lateral image acquisition, and saved images must be sent to storage to prevent the patient needing post-operative imaging in the radiology department.
- All staff present during image acquisition must be wearing appropriate lead protection. It is useful to have a supply available to those who are required to wear surgical gloves and gowns so that they can put these on prior to donning the surgical garments (**Figure 10.2a**).
- Maintain minimal distance between detector and patient to reduce air gap, magnification, skin dose and scatter. It will also increase the field of view, important when carrying out some procedures, and improve image quality. This is important to remember when moving from an AP/PA to lateral position.
- Make sure that the viewing monitors are adjusted for optimum contrast and brightness.
- Begin imaging on half dose and only change from this if the image quality is unsatisfactory. If the above recommendations have been implemented and do not improve image quality, it may be necessary to select digital spot mode but remember that this leads to a much higher dose.

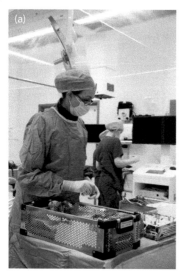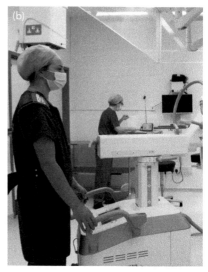

Figure 10.2 (a) Scrub nurse with lead protection, including thyroid shield, under surgical garments and (b) radiographer in theatre attire.

Infection Control

- The radiographer will need to wear theatre attire when entering theatre. This will comprise surgical scrubs, theatre cap, surgical mask and theatre shoes (**Figure 10.2b**).
- It is good practice to cover the detector and the X-ray tube head to ensure no fluid encroachment into the equipment if underneath the table.
- When the C-arm is in the sterile field, the scrub nurse will cover it with sterile drapes.

ORTHOPAEDIC SURGERY

Manipulation under Anaesthetic and Open Reduction Internal Fixation on Extremities

Manipulation under anaesthetic (MUA) does not involve open surgery and is used if a fracture is likely to be stable once reduced. Open reduction internal fixation (ORIF) requires the surgeon to insert a stabilisation device at the fracture site if it is felt that the fracture will be unstable following reduction.

There are many different forms of fixation devices, with some examples outlined in **Table 10.1**. Despite the method for reducing the fracture to achieve normal bone alignment or the stabilisation device used, the imaging technique is the same.

Table 10.1 Examples of different orthopaedic trauma procedures.

Procedure	Examples of fracture type being treated
Femoral head replacement Cancellous hip screws Dynamic hip screw (DHS) Gamma nail Dynamic condylar screw	Fracture of the femoral neck Slipped upper femoral epiphysis (SUFE)
Kirschner wire (K-wire) (**Figure 10.3a**) Pin and plate fixation (**Figure 10.3b**)	Simple extremity fracture Salter Harris fracture
Illizarov external fixator Taylor spatial frame Intramedullary nail fixation	Open or complex fractures Fractures with significant soft tissue involvement Closed fractures of the tibia or femur
Distal volaris radius plate (**Figure 10.3c**)	Intra-articular comminuted distal radial fractures
Tension band wiring (**Figure 10.3d**)	Olecranon and patella fracture/ displacement following trauma
Syndesmotic screw fixation	Syndesmosis injury to the ankle

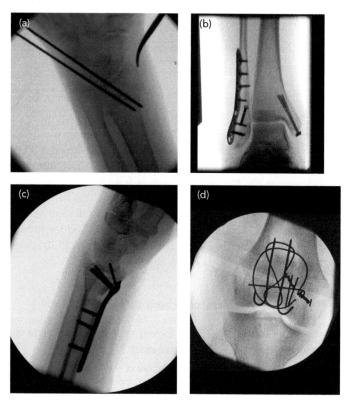

Figure 10.3 Examples of internal fixation devices: (a) K-wire in radius; (b) pin and plate fixation in a fibula; (c) distal volaris radius plate in radius; (d) tension band wiring of a patella.

Technique for MUA and ORIF

- The patient is usually supine on the table.
- How the mobile fluoroscopy machine is positioned depends on the surgery site. For lower limb surgery it is likely to be on the opposite side to that being operated on, whereas for upper limb surgery it will be on the same side. The surgeon must not operate directly over the detector, as it can easily be damaged. An arm board must be used for upper limb surgery (Figure 10.1b).

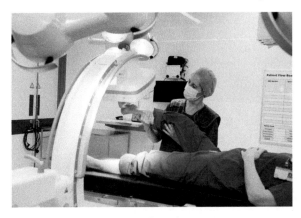

Figure 10.4 Surgeon rotating limb into lateral position.

- The surgeon may turn the limb during the procedure so be careful not to expose the surgeon's hands if they are holding the limb during screening (**Figure 10.4**). Occasionally the machine may need moving. Do this with care so that you do not desterilise the area.
- Positioning of a child on the theatre table is key to being able to obtain diagnostic images, as their limbs are unlikely to extend beyond the edge of the table. Screening through the table is possible but leads to a higher dose and possible artefacts. Placing the child close to the edge of the table will allow the arm board to be used for both upper and lower limb surgery and the area of interest to be placed close to the centre of the detector.

Dynamic Hip Screw or Cannulated Screws

A neck-of-femur fracture is generally surgically treated with fixation and the type of surgery will depend upon the type of fracture. Either a dynamic hip screw (DHS) or cannulated screws will be used (**Figure 10.5**), with a single cannulated screw also being used to fix a slipped upper femoral epiphysis (SUFE) in a child. DHS surgery consists of inserting a lag screw through a metal sleeve into the femoral head to increase compression at a displaced fracture site. A side plate is attached to the metal sleeve and fixed to the lateral femoral

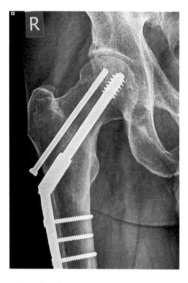

Figure 10.5 AP hip image demonstrating a DHS and a single cannulated screw.

cortex. Weight bearing causes dynamic compression of the fracture and the shaft of the screw slides down the sleeve, maintaining fracture reduction. Cannulated screws are inserted across a fracture that is undisplaced or impacted, or through the epiphysis if a SUFE is being treated. The aim of surgery is to stabilise the fracture site, allowing early mobilisation, preventing the complications of bed rest in older patients, giving the hip joint stability, increasing movement and reducing pain. The fluoroscopic technique is the same for each of these procedures.

Technique for DHS or Cannulated Screws

- The patient will be positioned supine on the table with the unaffected leg flexed at the hip and abducted (**Figure 10.6**).
- When positioning the mobile fluoroscopy machine, you will need effective communication with the team to ensure that the patient is positioned correctly so that you can achieve a true lateral image (**Figure 10.7**). This may require the patient's unaffected leg to be abducted slightly further. Often, externally rotating the lower leg will help to move the knee to enable the lateral image.
- Be mindful that often such patients will have been given a spinal epidural rather than a general anaesthetic so will be conscious and aware of their surroundings and background conversations.

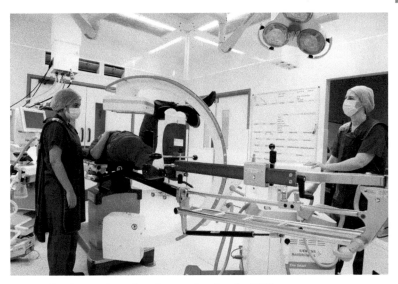

Figure 10.6 Positioning of machine and patient for DHS surgery.

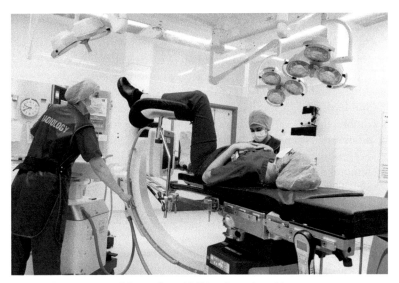

Figure 10.7 Rotation of C-arm from AP/PA to lateral position.

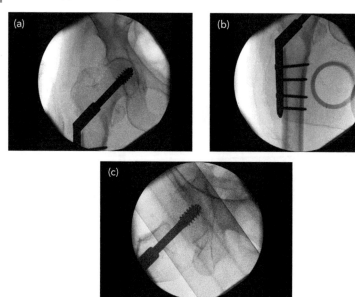

Figure 10.8 Images taken during DHS surgery: (a) AP/PA hip; (b) AP/PA proximal femur demonstrating plate; (c) lateral hip.

- Imaging will be required immediately to assist the surgeon with reducing the fracture to a satisfactory position.
- AP/PA and lateral images of the affected hip are required. Once you have taken your first images and you are happy with your mobile fluoroscopy machine position, lock the foot brake. Minor adjustments can be made using the individual locks.
- Screening will take place while the guidewire is inserted into the femoral neck and then during positioning of the lag screw and attachment of the side plate.
- Unless otherwise stated, three final images should be saved and sent to storage: an AP/PA of the hip to include the hip joint (**Figure 10.8a**), AP/PA of the plate on the proximal femur (**Figure 10.8b**) and a lateral of the hip and neck of femur (**Figure 10.8c**). Make sure this includes the hip joint and that the detector is as close as possible to the patient so that you maximise the field of view.

Hip Arthroscopy or Hip Arthrogram

Minimally invasive hip arthroscopy helps diagnose and treat some hip conditions and has a shorter recovery time than open surgery. A small incision is made and an arthroscope is inserted into the joint. The arthroscope contains a fibreoptic video camera that transmits images to a large monitor. Very thin surgical instruments can be inserted through small incisions to remove lose bone fragments, repair damaged cartilage or ligaments, or remove scar tissue. Arthroscopy is also performed in other joints, such as the knee and the shoulder, but fluoroscopy is not often used to support this surgery. A similar procedure is a hip arthrogram (**Figure 10.9**), which is carried out in theatre on a child as an investigative procedure prior to hip dysplasia surgery. A contrast agent is injected instead of air or fluid.

Technique for Hip Arthroscopy or Hip Arthrogram

- The patient will be positioned supine with legs extended and abducted.
- The surgeon will move the hip and may inject air or fluid into the joint. Screening will be required during this movement and only on the request of the surgeon. After applying manual traction, the surgeon may need a static image to confirm the presence of a vacuum crescent sign. If a hip arthrogram is being performed, a contrast agent will be injected at this point.

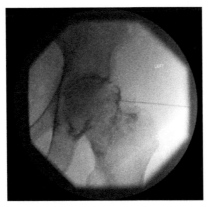

Figure 10.9 Intra-operative image demonstrating a hip arthrogram.

Proximal Femoral Nailing Anti-rotation

Proximal femoral nailing anti-rotation (PFNA) surgery is insertion of an intramedullary (IM) nail to femoral trochanteric or intertrochanteric fractures in osteoporotic patients (**Figure 10.10**). In addition, it can be used for femoral shaft fractures where femoral neck fractures are likely to occur in the future. It can also be performed in children who may have reduced bone density leading to pathological fractures. A PFNA's properties facilitate compaction of the cancellous bone, which in turn compacts the fracture site. It also reduces rotational movement and displacement and increases stability, allowing the patient to weight bear sooner.

Technique for PFNA

- The patient is positioned in the same way as for a DHS.
- The mobile fluoroscopy machine must be set up in such a way that it can move up and down the femur with ease and a true lateral image of the affected hip and the remainder of the femur can be achieved.
- Imaging in the AP/PA and lateral planes will be required immediately to assist the surgeon with reducing the fracture into a satisfactory position before insertion of a femoral guidewire with fluoroscopy guidance.

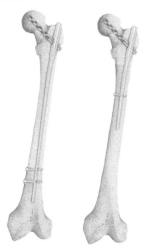

Figure 10.10 Long and short PFNAs (green denotes the fracture location).

- When imaging the distal nail, the central ray must be perpendicular to the hole drilled in the nail, seen as a circle rather than an oval (**Figure 10.11**). If it appears as an oval, adjust the angulation of the C-arm. This helps the surgeon identify the location for skin incision and placement of the distal locking screw.
- AP/PA and lateral images of the whole nail must be saved (**Figure 10.12**).

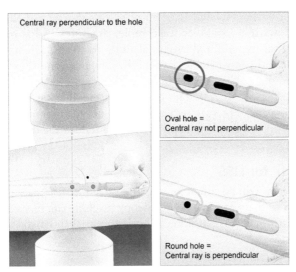

Figure 10.11 Distal locking hole demonstrating correct circle and incorrect oval.

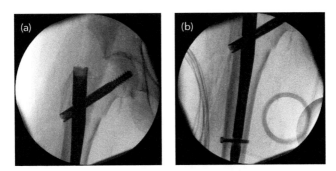

Figure 10.12 AP/PA images taken during PFNA surgery of (a) proximal nail and (b) distal nail.

Less Invasive Stabilisation System Plating of Femur

Less invasive stabilisation system (LISS) plating is a minimally invasive extramedullary internal fixation method commonly used to treat comminuted and often intra-articular fractures of long bones. As it is minimally invasive, there is less soft tissue damage or reduction in bone integrity. The surgical site is smaller, providing faster healing and allowing the patient to remain in hospital for a shorter period.

LISS allows more stability for complex fractures and is most used to treat distal femoral and proximal tibial fractures. Locking screws are fixed into the most stable parts of the long bone and these are connected by a plate. This leaves the most fragmented section of the bone untouched (**Figure 10.13**). The patient can mobilise faster than with other alternatives. Fracture reduction is not necessary prior to fixation; however, some surgeons will still attempt to reduce the fractures prior to fixation.

Technique for LISS

- The patient will be supine on the table.
- Make sure that the mobile fluoroscopy machine can be easily moved to enable visualisation of both proximal and distal aspects

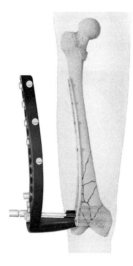

Figure 10.13 Diagram of the LISS fixation device.

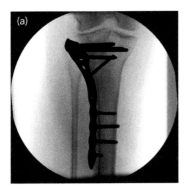 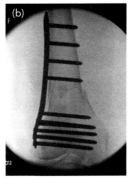

Figure 10.14 AP intra-operative image of (a) tibial LISS and (b) femoral LISS.

of the plating device in the AP/PA position and allow easy rotation of the C-arm into the lateral position.

- If the detector is below the patient, rotation to achieve a lateral projection will mean that the C-arm is over the table. The surgeon will raise and hold the sterile drape to maintain sterility of the operation site. It is likely that the detector, X-ray tube and C-arm will have already been draped.
- Unless otherwise stated, final images to be sent to storage should include AP/PA and lateral images to include the distal plate, fracture and adjacent joint space and the proximal plate (**Figure 10.14**).

Intramedullary Nailing of Long Bone Shaft Fractures

An IM nail is a method of internal fixation used to provide stability to long bone shaft fractures and is the preferred treatment of choice for fractures of the femoral shaft. The procedure is like a PFNA but does not have the femoral neck component and can be used on any long bone. Fracture healing is improved due to the lack of movement at the fracture site, and there is no resultant shortening of the affected limb. In treatment of lower limb fractures, the IM nail enables early weight bearing, which in turn increases bone growth and fracture healing. When fixing tibial shaft fractures, the surgeon may operate with the leg flexed around 15°. In this instance, the angle of the C-arm should be adjusted so that the central ray is perpendicular to the long axis of the tibia (**Figure 10.15**).

The IM nail is inserted into the medullary cavity of the long bone after placement of a guidewire under fluoroscopy control. The position of the guidewire is key to ensuring the nail is inserted correctly, and the surgeon will require visualisation of the distal aspect in both AP/PA and lateral planes. Once the nail is inserted, proximal and distal interlocking screws will be used to secure the nail in place. Again, the surgeon will need to do this under fluoroscopy control, so the mobile fluoroscopy machine needs to be positioned so that you can easily move along the shaft of the bone as well as rotate the C-arm into AP/PA and lateral positions.

Technique for IM Nail

- The imaging technique is the same as that for PFNA.
- Images of the proximal and distal nail must be saved in both planes (**Figure 10.16**).

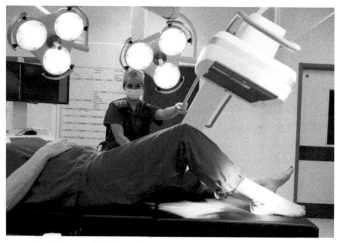

Figure 10.15 Angulation of C-arm to reflect knee flexion for tibial nailing.

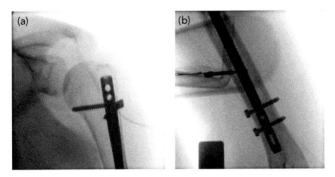

Figure 10.16 Intra-operative AP/PA humerus images to demonstrate (a) proximal nail and (b) distal nail.

Proximal Humeral Internal Locking Osteosynthesis System

Although the majority of undisplaced fractures through the proximal humerus are treated conservatively, patients with displaced (**Figure 10.17**) or comminuted fractures are most likely to require surgery using a locking plate called a proximal humeral internal locking (PHILOS) osteosynthesis system.[2] The aim is to achieve a painless and functional shoulder. Surgery is normally performed with the patient in a 'beach-chair' position (**Figure 10.18**).

Technique for PHILOS

- Although the patient does appear to be sitting up, they will be under general anaesthesia for this procedure.
- It is usual for the detector to be underneath the table and as close to the patient as possible. As the patient will be approached with the C-arm angulated, it is important to be careful and maintain patient safety when manoeuvring into position.
- To achieve a lateral image, do not adjust the position of the mobile fluoroscopy machine; the surgeon will manipulate the shoulder to demonstrate this position.
- Unless otherwise stated, one AP/PA and one lateral image should be sent to storage.

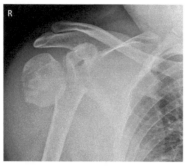

Figure 10.17 AP shoulder image demonstrating a displaced fracture.

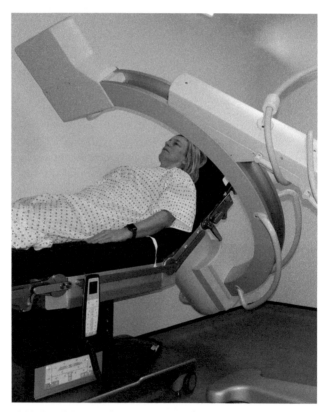

Figure 10.18 PHILOS procedure demonstrating the positions of both the patient and the mobile fluoroscopy machine.

Ilizarov or Taylor Spatial Frame

The Ilizarov and Taylor spatial frames are cylindrical external fixation devices for treating limb-lengthening discrepancies caused by congenital deformities or complex fractures.[3] They can be used separately or can be combined for more complicated fractures (**Figure 10.19**). K-wires are passed through the skin into the bones and fixed to external rings, which are connected to each other by rods. By making fine adjustments, the Ilizarov frame corrects longitudinal discrepancies, whereas the Taylor spatial frame uses oblique rods to correct angular deformities.

Technique for Ilizarov and Taylor Spatial Frames

- The imaging procedure is like the LISS procedure, but it is important to remember the protrusion of the wires when moving between AP/PA and lateral positions, as it is very easy for them to catch upon the C-arm.

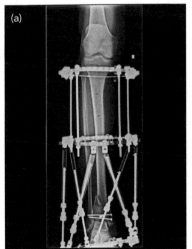 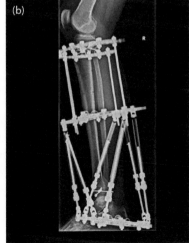

Figure 10.19 (a) AP and (b) lateral tibia and fibula images demonstrating combined Ilizarov (proximal) and Taylor spatial frame (distal).

Joint Injections

Pain lists are carried out in theatre for patients with chronic joint pain. An injection of local anaesthetic and steroid direct into the affected joint reduces inflammation and swelling and provides some level of pain relief for a period of time. Injections may be repeated every 3 months.

Technique for Joint Injection

- The patient will be either supine or prone depending on the joint being injected and will be awake throughout the procedure.
- A local anaesthetic will be injected into the skin prior to a needle being inserted into the joint and the injection taking place (**Figure 10.20**).
- The surgeon is likely to rotate the limb between projections, but it may be beneficial to ask if rotation of the C-arm will be needed before positioning the mobile fluoroscopy machine.

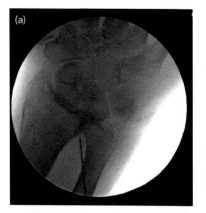 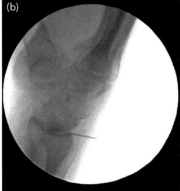

Figure 10.20 (a) AP/PA and (b) lateral wrist images demonstrating needle placement for joint injection.

NEUROSURGERY

Microdiscectomy and Laminectomy

Microdiscectomy and laminectomy procedures are carried out to relieve the spinal nerve impingement often caused by lumbar disc herniation.[4] Microdiscectomy involves removing the herniated disc material and occasionally a small portion of bone from around the nerve root to reduce the impingement on the nerve (**Figure 10.21**),

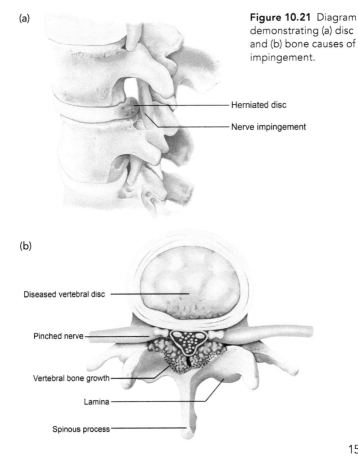

(a)

Figure 10.21 Diagram demonstrating (a) disc and (b) bone causes of impingement.

Herniated disc

Nerve impingement

(b)

Diseased vertebral disc

Pinched nerve

Vertebral bone growth

Lamina

Spinous process

whereas laminectomy improves the aperture of the neural foramina by removing part of the lamina and occasionally trimming the facet joints (**Figure 10.22**).

Technique for Microdiscectomy and Laminectomy

- The patient is prone and may be positioned on special padding or supports, such as a Wilson frame, to create flexion in the spine.
- It may only be possible to achieve lateral images. Rotating the C-arm over the patient will most likely be preferred but check before the machine is draped and sterile. The X-ray tube should be on top with the detector at the bottom before rotating the C-arm over the patient (**Figure 10.23**). Occasionally, oblique or PA images may be required.

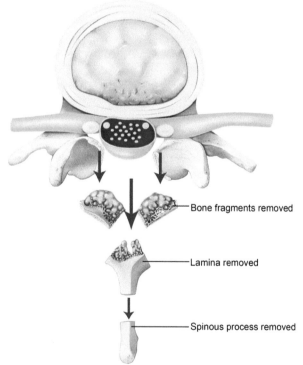

Bone fragments removed

Lamina removed

Spinous process removed

Figure 10.22 Diagram of vertebral body demonstrating laminectomy procedure.

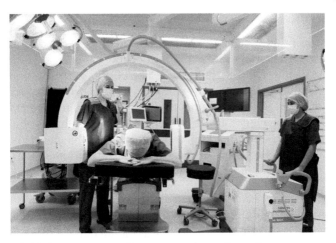

Figure 10.23 Demonstration of C-arm rotated over the patient.

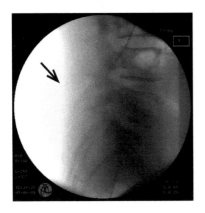

Figure 10.24 Intra-operative lateral lumbar spine image demonstrating placements of needle to identify level of surgery.

■ The surgeon will place a needle in the skin under fluoroscopy control to demonstrate the spinal level at which they will operate before they commence the procedure under sterile conditions (**Figure 10.24**).

■ Further imaging may be required during the surgery, and you will be advised if this is the case. It is normal to move the mobile fluoroscopy machine out of the way of the surgeon when not screening, moving it up or down the patient's body so that it can be moved easily back into place when needed.

Posterior Lumbar Interbody Fusion

A posterior lumbar interbody fusion (PLIF) is performed to fuse together vertebral bodies by the introduction of a bone graft or an implant such as a PEEK spinal cage. The PLIF procedure commences with a laminectomy at the affected level with the trimming of part or all of the facet joints and removal of the affected intervertebral disc. Pedicle screws (**Figure 10.25**) are inserted into the bones above and below to stabilise the disc level and cages filled with bone are inserted into the disc space to support fusion of the vertebral bodies. This can be quite a lengthy process and you will be required to obtain images throughout the placement of the pedicle screws.

Technique for PLIF

- The imaging technique is the same as for microdiscectomy and laminectomy.
- In between screening, see if the surgeon wants the mobile fluoroscopy machine moved towards the head of the patient.

Anterior Cervical Discectomy and Fusion

An anterior cervical discectomy and fusion (ACDF) fuses together cervical vertebrae to relieve pressure on the spinal cord and/or its nerves from an imposing disc. The procedure is performed through an incision on the anterior aspect of the neck (**Figure 10.26**). One or more intervertebral discs are removed along with any other small bony fragments, which may lead to impingement on the spinal nerve. A spacer bone graft is inserted into the cleared space and a plate is then screwed into place to allow fusion to take place.

Technique for ACDF

- The imaging technique is the same as for microdiscectomy and laminectomy, but the patient will be supine and ideally the surgeon will have positioned them so that their shoulders are as low as possible, and you are able to visualise as much of the cervical spine as possible.

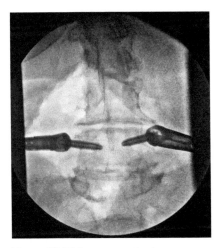

Figure 10.25 Intra-operative image of lumbar spine pedicle screw insertion.

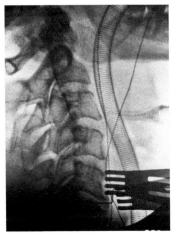

Figure 10.26 Intra-operative lateral cervical spine image taken during ACDF.

Scoliosis Surgery: Spinal Traction and Posterior Spinal Instrumentation and Fusion

In a paediatric setting, PLIF surgery does occur; however, posterior spinal instrumentation and fusion (PSIF) is more common as a way to correct curvatures of the spine. Scoliosis affects between 2 and 3% of the population with adolescent idiopathic scoliosis, with a Cobb angle greater than 10°, affecting between 0.93 and 12% of the population worldwide.[5] It affects females more than males.[5] PSIF surgery usually takes place once the patient has almost reached their full growth potential although this may vary between specialists.

Prior to the PSIF taking place, a radiographer may need to attend the theatre to acquire an image of the whole spine (AP) while the surgeon applies traction to stretch the spine prior to the PSIF procedure. In children, this may be done under anaesthetic for compliance. The images will help the surgeon ascertain the degree of flexibility the spine has and determine the level of surgery.

Technique for Spinal Traction

- Patient position is supine on the operating table with a large detector underneath the patient's spine.
- The mobile X-ray machine is centred and collimated to include the area of interest, prior to applying traction and as confirmed by the surgeon.
- Carry out a test run to ensure everyone is aware of their role and that the image detector and collimation still cover the area of interest once traction is applied.
- Make final adjustments and then acquire an image.

Technique for PSIF

- Patient position is prone on the operating table.
- Most surgeons prefer the C-arm to rotate over the patient to demonstrate the neck in a lateral aspect, but this is not always the case, and it is good practice to ask what the surgeon requires before the mobile fluoroscopy machine is draped and sterile.
- At the start of the case the surgeon may require the radiographer to be present to perform a level check. This enables them to assess the level at which they will be performing surgery.
- In the case of scoliosis, and due to the varied position of the vertebra, the radiographer will often be required to adjust the C-arm on a frequent basis. This will facilitate the surgeon in viewing the vertebra in a PA/AP position so that they can clearly see the pedicles. Good visualisation of the pedicles is paramount, as this will enable the surgeon to decide if the pedicles are suitable and allow for placement of the pedicle screws (**Figure 10.27**). The radiographer will be required to screen in both AP/PA and lateral planes while the screws are being positioned. Once the pedicle screws are in place the surgeon will request a final AP/PA and lateral check of all screws; then a rod can be attached to enable the curvature to be reduced.

Facet Joint Injection

The facet joints are located on the back of the spine, one on each side of each vertebra, and comprise the two opposing surfaces of neighbouring vertebrae, which are separated by a thin layer of cartilage and

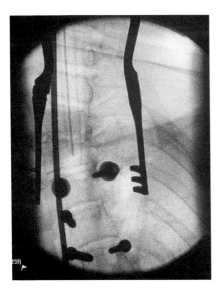

Figure 10.27 Intra-operative image of pedicle screws being inserted.

surrounded by a fluid-filled capsule. They not only provide stability but also allow the spine to bend and twist. Facet joint injections involve injecting into the capsule or the soft tissues surrounding the joints.[6] Diagnostic injections, or nerve blocks, are used to determine if the facet joint is the source of pain. Therapeutic injections are used to relieve pain and may require repeating. The patient will be awake for this procedure, but it is usually performed in the theatre environment due to patient recovery time requirements.

Technique for Facet Joint Injections

- If the thoracic or lumbar region is to be imaged, the patient will be prone (**Figure 10.28**); however, the cervical region usually requires the patient to be in the supine position.
- A local anaesthetic is initially injected at the relevant level prior to the surgeon inserting a needle into the facet joint and injecting a contrast solution to assist in needle placement. An injection of local anaesthetic and steroid is then made into the facet joint.
- Screen at the request of the surgeon and use the laser light, if available, to centre the required body part in the middle of the field of view, collimating appropriately.

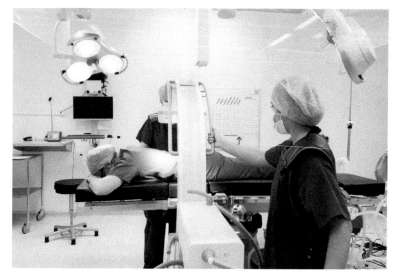

Figure 10.28 Position of mobile fluoroscopy machine for facet joint injections.

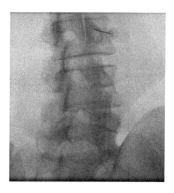

Figure 10.29 Needle inserted into L2/L3 left facet with fluoroscopic guidance.

- Begin imaging on half dose and only change from this if the image quality is unsatisfactory, with digital spot mode being a last resort.
- Facet joint injections usually only require AP/PA images to guide the insertion of the needle (**Figure 10.29**); however, the surgeon may occasionally require a lateral image.
- Send images to storage as requested by the surgeon.

Nerve Root Injections

Nerve root injections are a tool used to diagnose patients with chronic neuropathic pain – that is, nerve pain that has been caused by irritation, damage or the destruction of nerves – in the legs. The injections limit the brain's ability to interpret pain through a mixture of local anaesthetic and steroids being injected directly into a nerve or the nerve bundle to inhibit its functionality.

Technique for Nerve Root Injections

- The patient and mobile fluoroscopy machine are positioned as for facet joint injections; however, it is worth noting that some surgeons will position the patient on their side (**Figure 10.30**).
- Imaging guidance will be required in the AP/PA position and in the lateral position.
- The procedure follows the same steps as facet injections, but the anaesthetic and steroid mix is injected into a nerve root as opposed to the facet joint.
- The image demonstrating contrast with the correct needle placement is always a good image to save for documentation.

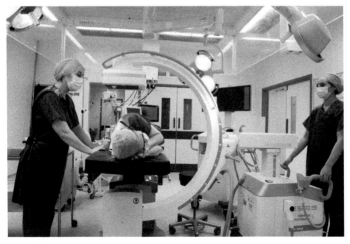

Figure 10.30 Patient positioned on their side for nerve root injection.

Trigeminal Nerve Block or Rhizotomy

Trigeminal pain comes from one or more branches of the trigeminal nerve, the main carrier of sensory information from the face to the brain (**Figure 10.31**). Patients may have a nerve block or a rhizotomy.[7] A nerve block involves injecting anaesthetic into the affected nerve whereas a rhizotomy involves inserting a needle into the nerve bundle to damage it. Both prevent signals from being transmitted to the brain.

Technique for Trigeminal Nerve Block or Rhizotomy

- Most surgeons prefer the C-arm to rotate over the patient for the lateral image, but it is good practice to ask the surgeon before sterile drapes are in place.
- There will be an air gap, causing magnification. Try to reduce this by having the detector as close to the area being imaged as possible and collimate using the iris collimator.
- Both AP/PA and lateral images are needed to ensure that the needle is correctly sited.
- Send images to storage as requested by the surgeon.

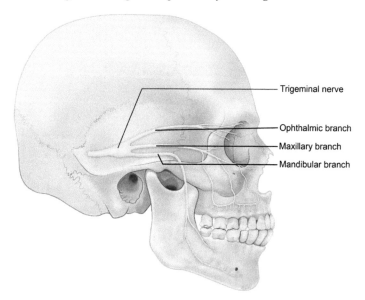

Figure 10.31 Location of the trigeminal nerve.

UROLOGY

Stent Insertion/Removal

A stent is a thin tube placed inside the ureter to allow urine to pass into the bladder if an obstruction has been identified (**Figure 10.32**). Common causes of obstruction are renal stones, ureteric strictures and post-surgery inflammation. A cystoscope is passed into the bladder to see the ureteric opening, and the stent is inserted via the urethra and bladder into the ureter.

Technique for Stent Insertion/Removal

■ The patient will have a general or a spinal anaesthetic and be supine.
■ Once positioned over the ureter, align the mobile fluoroscopy machine wheels to enable smooth steering when imaging the length of the ureter as required.

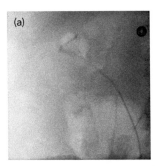 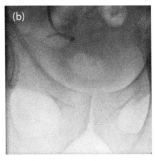

Figure 10.32 Intra-operative images obtained during stent placement demonstrating (a) proximal stent within kidney; (b) distal stent within bladder.

Percutaneous Nephrolithotomy

A percutaneous nephrolithotomy (PCNL) is a procedure to remove kidney stones. A catheter is passed through the urethra and into the kidney or upper ureter to enable contrast enhancement to be performed throughout the procedure. When the kidney is enhanced with contrast, the surgeon will puncture the skin of the abdomen and create a tract with a series of wires and dilators. They will then pass a nephroscope through the sheath, which has been placed to maintain the tract so that the stones can be seen (**Figure 10.33**). Other instruments can be inserted through the same tract and the stones are either removed or broken up using high-frequency sound waves. An irrigation system, incorporated into the nephroscope, washes away stone fragments, so it is important to ensure that water does not come into contact with the detector.

A nephrostomy tube is then passed through the tract and into the kidney to assist with drainage (**Figure 10.34**). The tube will be removed after a few days if a contrast injection confirms that the ureter is not blocked. Screening will be required throughout the procedure.

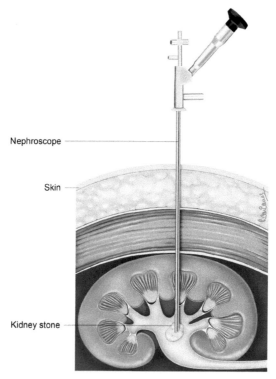

Nephroscope

Skin

Kidney stone

Figure 10.33 Insertion of nephroscope into the kidney.

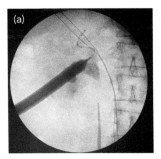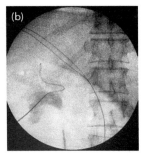

Figure 10.34 Intra-operative PCNL contrast-enhanced images demonstrating (a) nephrostomy tract; (b) nephrostomy tube.

Technique for PCNL

- The patient will be anaesthetised and will be turned into a prone oblique position after passing the catheter through the urethra into the kidney.
- Use the iris collimator unless the whole urinary tract is needed, in which case the lateral collimators will need to be used.
- If a radiologist is involved, attach the foot pedal and allow them to screen when required. As the radiologist will be directing radiation, you will need to be mindful of staff entering the operating theatre without lead coats.
- Once the radiologist has completed their part of the procedure, disconnect the foot pedal. You will provide screening for the rest of the examination.

Ureteroscopy with or without Lithotripsy

A ureteroscopy is an upper urinary tract endoscopy that is commonly performed with an endoscope passed through the urethra and bladder and then into the ureter. Ureteral stones almost always originate in the kidneys but can continue to grow once lodged in the ureter. Like the stent insertion procedure, ureteroscopy is performed under general or spinal anaesthetic with the patient remaining in the supine position. Images are acquired while contrast is injected through the catheter directly into the ureter (**Figure 10.35**). Any stones, even those that are radiolucent, and any strictures or tortuosities that may not

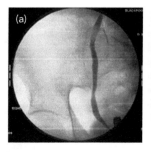 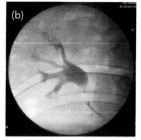

Figure 10.35 Images acquired during contrast injection demonstrating (a) distal ureter; (b) proximal ureter.

be visualised easily on other studies are clearly demonstrated. Small stones can be removed during ureteroscopy but larger stones may need to be fragmented first using lithotripsy. This involves sending ultrasound shock waves transcutaneously to break down the stone into smaller pieces, which can then be removed. When the ureteroscopy is complete, internal ureteral stents are commonly placed to ensure drainage and to facilitate healing.

Technique for Ureteroscopy

- The imaging technique is the same as for stent insertion/removal.

VASCULAR IMAGING

Emergency Peripheral Angiography

Emergency angiography is most likely to occur in a theatre environment. It is used to assess patency of vessels during surgery for complex and often open fractures or when bypass grafting is required. Mobile fluoroscopy units used for vascular work tend to have a larger detector and are more powerful due to the need for rapid image acquisition. Subtraction angiography should also be possible. An image referred to as a 'mask' is acquired prior to contrast injection and this is used to subtract non-useful information from the contrast-enhanced images (**Figure 10.36a**) leaving only the vascular anatomy visible (**Figure 10.36b**). Continuous flow through the vessels is visualised in the subtracted mode, showing the patency and any pathology of the affected vessel. Techniques such as 'road mapping' should also be available, where the best image following injection of contrast media is used and superimposed on the dynamic image to help with the positioning of guidewires and catheters.

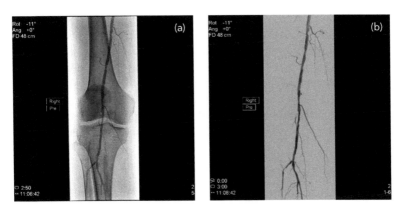

Figure 10.36 Images demonstrating the popliteal artery: (a) native image; (b) subtracted image.

Technique for Emergency Peripheral Angiography

- The patient will be supine during the procedure. It is important to make sure that the patient is positioned so that the required range of movement of the machine can be achieved with ease.

- An arterial catheter will be inserted, usually by Seldinger technique as described in *Clark's Procedures in Diagnostic Imaging: A System-Based Approach*.[8]

- Use the laser light, if available, to centre the required body part, to include the bone and adjacent arteries, in the middle of the field of view, collimating appropriately.

- If subtraction angiography is required, the 'mask' image must be obtained prior to the injection of contrast. Screening may be needed before, during and after contrast injection with 2–3 frames per second (fps) above the knee and 1 fps for the run-off series below the knee. Dedicated foot images are often undertaken and may require some angulation of the C-arm.

- Pulsed fluoroscopy should be used to minimise the dose, as long screening times are sometimes required.

- Copper filters, if available, and close collimation will improve image quality.

Endovascular Aneurysm Repair

Endovascular aneurysm repair (EVAR) is a minimally invasive procedure carried out to repair an aortic aneurysm. It is also referred to as thoracic EVAR (TEVAR) if the aneurysm is in the thoracic aorta. A custom-made graft, comprising a fabric-covered mesh stent, is inserted into the aorta at the level of the aneurysm through the groin. This expands, protecting the aorta from rupture. A contralateral stent limb is inserted in the base of the main stent body from the opposite femoral artery. The limbs of the EVAR stents help to protect the femoral vessels if the aneurysm extends into them and anchors the stents in position.

Technique for EVAR

- The imaging technique is the same as for emergency peripheral angiography.

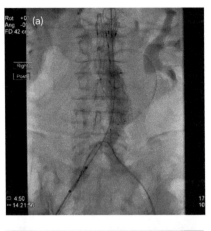

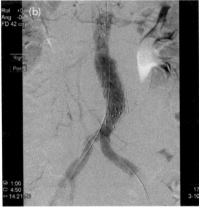

Figure 10.37 Images demonstrating (a) EVAR stent at site of abdominal aortic aneurysm; (b) subtracted image.

- Pre-procedural angiograms will be conducted before the surgeon positions the EVAR stent, and multiple angiogram runs may be required during the procedure.
- A post-procedural angiogram will be required to demonstrate that there are no leaks that compromise the integrity of the repair and are life threatening (**Figure 10.37**). Further angioplasty ballooning of the stents may be required if any endoleaks are demonstrated.

CARDIAC PACING

Pacing can be a temporary or a permanent solution to a cardiac problem. A temporary pacemaker can be inserted to treat an immediately life-threatening condition and remains in situ until that condition is treated or a permanent pacemaker can be inserted. There are several ways of temporarily pacing the heart:

- transvenous pacing, the most common procedure, involving a pacing lead being passed intravenously into the right atrium/ ventricle;
- external (transcutaneous) pacing, which is used in a peri-arrest or cardiac arrest;
- epicardial pacing, which involves ventricular and arterial pacing leads being attached to the pericardium.

Permanent pacemaker insertions are normally implanted transvenously in the left shoulder region and are generally done under local anaesthetic with conscious sedation. The standard pacemaker usually comes in two parts: the pacemaker generator housing the electronics and battery and placed in a pocket below the clavicle, and the pacemaker lead(s), long insulated wires that can sense intrinsic contraction of the heart chamber and stimulate contraction (pacing) when needed. Depending on the heart problem a specific type of pacemaker ranging from one to three leads may be used:

- single-chamber pacemaker: a single lead attached to one chamber of the heart (right ventricle);
- dual-chamber pacemaker: two leads attached to two chambers of the heart (right atrium and right ventricle);
- biventricular pacemaker: usually three leads; two are attached to the right and left ventricles and the third lead may or may not be inserted in the right atrium depending upon the heart rhythm.

Biventricular pacemakers are used in advanced heart failure and deliver two functions: an electrical stimulus similar to the single-/ dual-chamber pacemaker and/or a shock if they detect a dangerous rhythm. The latter is done by an implantable cardioverter defibrillator (ICD), also called a biventricular ICD.

Leadless pacemakers are much smaller than traditional pacemakers, being the size of a large pill. These are inserted via the femoral vein and attached to the inner wall of the right ventricle.

There is a risk of cardiac arrest during pacing procedures so be prepared to raise the detector, or move the machine, if possible, to give access to the chest for CPR.

Technique for Temporary Pacemaker Insertion

■ The patient is supine and venous access is gained via the internal jugular or femoral veins. A venogram is performed at a frame rate of 3–7.5 fps. The frame with the most vessel opacification is stored as a 'roadmap' image. This is used as the mask and subtracted from the subsequent dynamic fluoroscopy images.

■ A venous sheath is inserted, through which the lead is introduced into the right ventricle.

– From a femoral approach the lead is advanced to the right ventricle via the external iliac vein, the inferior vena cava, the right atrium and then through the tricuspid valve to the right ventricle.

– From a jugular approach the lead is advanced to the brachiocephalic vein, the superior vena cava, the right atrium and through the tricuspid valve to the right ventricle. Once in the right ventricle, the tip of the lead should point towards the left hip and be in contact with the endocardial tissue (**Figure 10.38**).

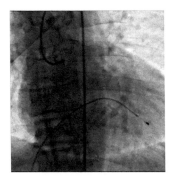

Figure 10.38 PA projection of the heart demonstrating a lead in the right ventricle apex with the tip pointing towards the left hip.

- Screening is needed during lead insertion with a low frame rate of 3–7.5 fps and careful collimation is needed to demonstrate the tip of the lead.
- A left anterior oblique (LAO) 30° or right anterior oblique (RAO) 30° projection may be used to confirm lead position.

Technique for Permanent Pacemaker Insertion

- Radiographically the procedure is the same as temporary pacemaker insertion. With fluoroscopic guidance in the PA projection, the left axillary or subclavian vein is cannulated and a sheath inserted. Depending on the type of pacemaker implanted, one, two or three venous access points are used for a single-chamber, dual-chamber or biventricular pacemaker, respectively.
- A single wire is positioned in the right ventricle via the superior vena cava.
- For a dual-chamber pacemaker another wire is introduced into the second sheath in the shoulder and advanced into the right atrium.
- For the biventricular pacemaker or implantable cardioverter defibrillator device, a lead is also placed into the left ventricle via a branch of the coronary sinus, which drains from the posterolateral aspect of the left ventricle.
- Using fluoroscopy, a LAO 30° or RAO 30° projection may be used to confirm position of the wires and generator (**Figure 10.39**).
- A final stored fluoroscopic run demonstrating the pacemaker leads and the generator is performed.

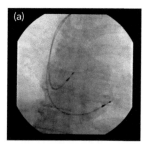 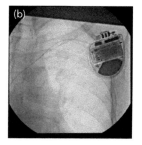

Figure 10.39 Fluoroscopic images demonstrating (a) lead position; (b) generator position.

GENERAL SURGERY

Endoscopic Retrograde Cholangiopancreatography

Endoscopic retrograde cholangiopancreatography (ERCP) is performed to diagnose and treat problems in the bile ducts, gallbladder, liver and pancreas. Often performed in a static fluoroscopy room under sedation, it may also be performed under general anaesthesia in a theatre suite. An endoscope is passed through the mouth and into the duodenum, close to the bile and pancreatic ducts. A catheter is passed into the biliary duct and contrast injected.

Technique for ERCP

- The patient is positioned on their left side initially and then may be turned prone to assist in passing the catheter into the biliary duct.
- Continuous screening will be needed so that the clinician can watch the progression of the endoscope and catheter, and then the introduction of contrast media as it flows through the biliary duct (**Figure 10.40a**).
- A stent may be placed into the bile duct if there is an obstruction (**Figure 10.40b**), allowing bile to drain freely and prevent jaundice.

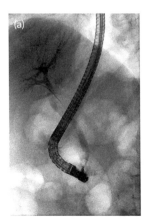
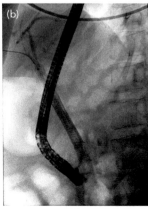

Figure 10.40 ERCP images demonstrating (a) filling of the biliary tree; (b) placement of a biliary stent.

Operative Cholangiogram

An operative cholangiogram, often referred to as an op chole, is performed to assess the biliary tree for gall stones during surgery for gallbladder removal. This is normally done laparoscopically. The surgeon will temporarily clip the cystic duct, inject contrast into it and then, with fluoroscopy guidance, view the contrast media as it travels through the biliary tree.

Technique for Operative Cholangiogram

- The patient will be positioned supine.
- Once the mobile fluoroscopy machine is in the right position, contrast will be injected and live screening will commence. Ensure that continuous radiation is selected, as this will be required when the contrast is injected.
- If the mobile fluoroscopy machine has a cine loop, then the images will be saved. If this option isn't available, then the last screen hold should be saved instead (**Figure 10.41**).

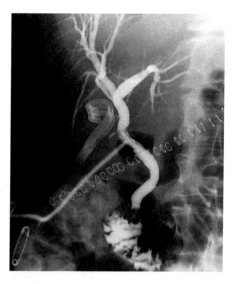

Figure 10.41 Image of biliary tree during an operative cholangiogram.

PROSTATE BRACHYTHERAPY

Brachytherapy involves the use of a temporary or permanent internal radiation source, in the form of seeds, to treat cancer, mainly of the prostate.

Technique for Prostate Brachytherapy

- The patient will be in the supine position on the operating table with the legs flexed at the hips and held in abduction with stirrups.
- The surgeon will pass thin needles through the perineum and into the prostate where the seeds will be released (**Figure 10.42**).

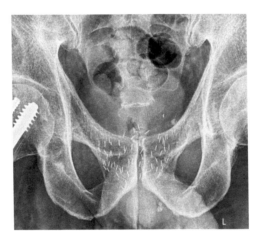

Figure 10.42 Demonstration of brachytherapy seeds on post-operative X-ray.

CHAPTER SUMMARY

- Always ensure identity and pregnancy checks have been completed and follow local procedures if the patient is already anaesthetised.
- It is best to have the detector above the patient; however, image quality can be affected if there is a large object–detector distance. The surgeon may prefer the detector to be below the patient for convenience and ease of access to the patient anatomy.
- Make sure all staff are wearing lead protection.
- Collimate to improve image quality and reduce dose.
- A laser light will help with correct centring of the equipment.
- Fluoroscopy must only be initiated on the request of the clinician.
- Make sure that the viewing monitors are adjusted for optimum contrast and brightness.
- Screen on half dose and only change from this if the image quality is unsatisfactory.
- Cover the detector and X-ray tube head if they are not draped, to ensure no fluid encroachment into the equipment.

REFERENCES

1. Martin, A.J. and Dodd, E. First steps into practice: the value of preceptorship. *Imaging and Oncology* 2020;**34**:34–39.

2. Fletcher, J.W.A., Windolf, M., Richards, G., Gueorguiev, B., Buschbaum, J. and Varga, P. Importance of locking plate positioning in proximal humeral fractures as predicted by computer simulations. *Journal of Orthopaedic Research* 2018;**37**:957–964.

3. Hosny, G.A. Limb lengthening history, evolution, complications and current concepts. *Journal of Orthopaedics and Traumatology* 2020;**21**(1):3.

4. Ahn, Y. Devices for minimally invasive microdiscectomy: current status and future prospects. *Expert Review of Medical Devices* 2020;**17**(2):131–138.

5. Sung, S. Chae, H.W., Lee, H.S., Kim, S., Kwon, J.W., Lee, S.B. et al. Incidence and surgery rate of idiopathic scoliosis: a nationwide database study. *International Journal of Environmental Research and Public Health*. 2021;**18**(15):8152.

6. Won, H., Yang, M. and Kim, Y. Facet joint injections for management of low back pain: a clinically focused review. *Anesthesia and Pain Medicine* 2020; **15**(1):8–18.

7. Jeyaraj, P. Efficiency and efficacy of real-time fluoroscopic image-guided percutaneous Gasserian glycerol rhizotomy (PGGR), for intractable cases of trigeminal neuralgia. *Journal of Maxillofacial and Oral Surgery* 2022;**21**:1053–1064.

8. Whitley, A.S., Dodgeon, J., Meadows, A., Cullingworth, J., Holmes, K., Jackson, M. et al. *Clark's Procedures in Diagnostic Imaging: A System-Based Approach*. Boca Raton: CRC Press, 2020.

INDEX

Note: page numbers in *italics* refer to figures.

For Product Safety Concerns and Information please contact our EU representative GPSR@taylorandfrancis.com Taylor & Francis Verlag GmbH, Kaufingerstraße 24, 80331 München, Germany

T - #0234 - 160425 - C200 - 198/129/10 - PB - 9781032147826 - Gloss Lamination